FIT FOR SPORT

FIT FOR SPORT

Improving Physical Health for Successful Safer Sport

by

TERRY MOULE, N.D., D.O.

Foreword by Daley Thompson

PATRICK STEPHENS LIMITED Wellingborough

First published in 1986

British Library Cataloguing in Publication Data
Moule, Terry

Fit for sport: a programme for getting the
most from the games that you play.
1. Physical fitness   2. Sports—Physiological
aspects
I. Title
613.71   RA776

ISBN 85059-846-X

*Patrick Stephens Limited is part of the
Thorsons Publishing Group*

Printed and bound in Great Britain
by The Garden City Press, Letchworth, Herts.

CONTENTS

FOREWORD

by

Daley Thompson

This book is quality reading in that it has valuable information that can and will benefit readers, be they engaged in sport or thinking about some kind of involvement. It shows a good comprehension as to the body's prerequisites before sport is undertaken and more importantly while it is being played.

Now that people have more leisure time on their hands they are playing more sport and taking more exercise. That, allied to a greater awareness of how the body works and functions can only lead to a healthier person with a more positive attitude and outlook.

When you do exercise you put your body under stress so wear and tear are part and parcel of the course. Everyone is liable to injury but if you go through the procedures properly the chances of continual aches and pains can be reduced.

Above all this book stresses that preparation is paramount and I like that.

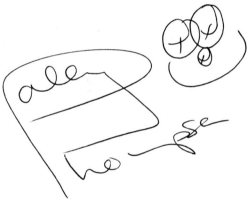

INTRODUCTION

At a time when there is a growing awareness of the fact that health is a matter of individual responsibility, there is a great shortage of information available to the public as to how to get the greatest benefit from sport, physical activity, and competitive team events. The common concept is that it is a good idea to play sport to keep fit, whereas in truth one should get fit in order to be able to play sport. If this basic approach is not used, then sport can be injurious and potentially detrimental to long-term health.

A prerequisite for playing any form of sport involving increased bodily activity is that the standard of a person's health is of a sufficiently high level to enable participation without producing damage or undue stress to the body. It is, therefore, important to understand the ground-rules for the achievement and maintenance of good health.

The human being is essentially designed to maintain normal health, so long as his environmental and living standards do not obstruct this natural ability. There are three areas where man can interfere with the normal function of the body, these being dietetically, structurally and psychologically. Any interference with any one of these will automatically produce some degree of malfunction in the others. It is important to look at each of these factors in greater detail.

The dietetic obstructive factor is of paramount importance, since the chemical intake of the body is critical if healthy muscle tone and tissue tone are to be maintained.

To understand what constitutes a sensible, balanced diet, one should first look at the type of food for which man's organism is designed. The slow digestive processes of the human intestinal tract, in particular, leads us to the conclusion that the bulk of the food intake should be of a fruit, salad and vegetable nature with a restriction on the amount of non-vegetarian proteins. An excessive intake of animal proteins, especially red meats, can produce a build-up of acid by-products within the body which, long term, can affect the organism's ability to perform to its full capacity. There has been a considerable tendency of late for sports persons to eat large quantities of animal proteins and this has led to an increase in the number of muscular problems.

It is important to eat efficiently: that means, only eat foods which have some value, and not 'junk foods', or ones which are of little significance dietetically. White flours, white sugars, tinned foods, processed foods, and foods which have been excessively cooked should all be regarded as belonging to this group, and should only be taken in minimal quantities. Fizzy drinks and cordials, etc, all of which contain a high quantity of processed sugars, should also be treated with some degree of circumspection.

Regularity is important in any form of dietary understanding, and every effort should be made to take meals at consistent intervals, particularly when trying to increase one's general physical abilities. Another potential area of problem is the hurried lunch or food eaten while on the move. Meals of this nature are not digested properly, rarely contain much of any value, and can produce such irritating side effects as indigestion and abdominal discomfort.

The necessity for the correct food intake cannot be over-emphasized: there is a lot of truth in the old saying: 'We are what we eat'. The question of specific dietary intake, and eating to produce certain physical results, is dealt with in detail in the first section of the book

The structural interference with normal function is the area where active involvement in sport becomes so important. Life is essentially to do with motion and mobility, and a lack of these produces a reduction in the efficiency of the body as a working unit. Civilization today tends to cause people to spend many hours sitting in cars, buses, trains, at desks or in armchairs, most of which have little or no relationship to the human shape. The effect of this sedentary existence is that the spine, which is critical if normal function is to be maintained, can become rigid, out of alignment, and even, in extreme cases, misshapen. To offset this problem, controlled exercise and activity is an absolute must.

It is important to realize that because of the relatively large amount of static time to which most bodies are subjected, it can be very detrimental to undertake sport only on a brief and intermittent basis, eg, one game of squash per week, and do nothing for the rest of the time. All sports have their inherent potential dangers, due to the various idiosyncrasies of how they are played, and these will be discussed further and in detail in the chapter relating to each specific sport. Over and above being involved in a sport itself, the necessity for regular daily exercise really cannot be overstated.

From the psychological point of view, stress and tension are factors of everyday life in the modern world. The physical effect of these is to produce related muscular tensions throughout the body, particularly in the neck and shoulders. Such tensions have the effect of reducing the ability of the body to function at its optimum level. Because of the close relationship between stress and muscular tension, releasing the physical tension has the reverse effect and helps to relieve the long-term effects of mental stress and trauma. This benefit yet again underlines the need for both regular and carefully selected exercise.

The approach to basic health outlined here is somewhat different from the usual line of 'let's train up from the base that we have got'. Since health is a normal state, what we are setting out to do is to take away those factors of everyday life which prevent this normality occurring. The more of these obstructions that can be removed, the greater the effect that training, coaching and specific exercise will have upon the body. These latter factors will always improve upon the basic ability of the individual in question, the important thing is to make sure that that basic ability is fully realized before undertaking the specific instruction necessary to improve technique.

There is another factor to be considered before undertaking any specific sport, and that is whether one is basically suited to the sport in question. Many people cause themselves discomfort, stress, and even embarrassment by attempting to take part in some form of sport or exercise for which they are totally unsuited. Body types are inherited, and one must select a suitable outlet for one's sporting inclinations. A 5 ft 4 in, fourteen-stone (196 lb) man is unlikely to achieve great success in playing basketball, but equally, the same man could well produce very good results in a sport such as rugby football.

An awareness of physical activity and the needs for it is, thank goodness, becoming much more common. Through the remainder of this book, it is hoped to show that sport need not entail excessive discomfort or long-term side effects — these being the result of poor training, poor preparation, and a total lack of understanding of the body's requirements to satisfactorily carry out a sporting role. An involvement in some form of sporting activity, subject to the right physical and mental approach, can only enhance the quality of life of the individual concerned.

ACKNOWLEDGEMENTS

I would like to express my thanks to a number of people who have made the writing of this book possible.

Firstly, I would like to thank Fatima Whitbread, Gerry Francis and Steve Redgrave for their kindness in posing for the exercise photographs, and also Daley Thompson for his interest in the book and for writing the Foreword. My particular thanks are due to Hilary Wilson, without whose high speed efforts at the typewriter keyboard none of my 'words of wisdom' would ever have reached the publishers on time.

I would also like to thank all those friends and fellow sportsmen who, over the years, have enabled me to become involved in sports medicine to the extent that I now am. Lastly, I would like to record my gratitude to my wife, without whose patience and understanding of my continued disappearance to every possible sporting venue, none of this would have been possible.

THE IMPORTANCE OF WHAT YOU EAT

It is impossible to contemplate undertaking regular physical activity without first making sure that our dietary intake is properly controlled and of a suitable nature to produce a healthy body. The food that we eat and what we drink has to be looked upon as building material that enables the body to chemically maintain and develop a good blood supply, good muscle tone and elasticity, and an active and responsive mind. As with building a house, if the material used is not of a sufficiently high quality, then the fabric will soon begin to show cracks and defects and, in many cases, the structure may even fall down.

The human body needs a balanced intake of a large number of vitamins, minerals, proteins, carbohydrates, fats, fibre, liquid etc. If any one or any number of these factors are not present in the diet, or if they are not presented in the proper way, then the ability of the organism to function will be reduced. The balance of these various factors — that is, what is eaten with what — is also very important and the nature of the source of these elements has a great effect on their subsequent usage.

For most effective usage of food and, therefore, maximum health, the art is to obtain the greatest possible amount of usable nutrition from the food with the least possible waste left over after the body's chemical processes have taken place. Whatever food we eat is processed by the body, anything of value taken from it, and the remainder has to be eliminated from within the body either via the kidneys and the urinary system, or through the intestinal tract, or the skin through sweating. It is obvious that the more efficiently these three eliminative functions work, then the greater the ability of the body to remove any waste product produced during the process of digestion and assimilation.

The digestive, assimilative and eliminative functions all require energy in order to be carried out, but only as much energy as necessary should be used for this: the more energy used for these functions, the less there is for the conscious activities, particularly strenuous activities such as sport and exercise. There is only one amount of energy available and, from this amount, the body has to control all the unconscious activities, as well as undertake day-to-day work, mental and physical activity and, of course, intensive activity under stress conditions. If the conscious activities, which will take precedence because of our own ability to determine what we do, cause a shortage of energy on the eliminative side, then obviously waste from the food we have eaten will not be fully eliminated. This causes a change in the body's chemistry and a build-up of acid waste matter which, in the long term, produces muscles which are less elastic and more prone to damage, joints prone to inflammation and ultimately such problems as fibrositis, rheumatism and arthritis.

In view of the foregoing, it is clearly preferable to use foods as near to their natural state as possible, as this is when the maximum usable contents are available. Processed foods, tinned foods and complicated preparations frequently contain a large amount of waste residue and a relatively small amount of usable nutritional material. At the same time, the more that foods are cooked and heated, the greater the nutritional value that is lost: raw foods and fresh fruits are to be encouraged at all times.

Shown here is a sensible, balanced diet which provides an adequate and balanced intake for anybody to carry on their normal way of life, but which will also raise their health level to a point where they can undertake considerable extra physical activity without causing problems of a chemical nature within the body. Lunch and evening meals may be transposed, but meals should not be missed out. If not really hungry, take small portions of each item. Drinks should not be taken with meals and only sufficient to quench the thirst.

Breakfast — select from:
1. Baked tomatoes on wholemeal toast and *Flora* or similar polyunsaturated margarine.
2. Muesli with soaked raisins and grated raw apple softened with apple juice or water.
3. Half grapefruit with fresh or stewed apple.
4. One or two slices of wholemeal toast and *Flora* with grated raw carrot.
5. Melon. Wholemeal crispbread and *Flora* with watercress and radishes.

Lunch
Large, varied raw salad with additional items selected from:
1. Ground or milled nuts. One or two wholemeal crispbread and *Flora*. Fresh or stewed apple to follow.
2. Nut meat, baked jacket potato. Half grapefruit to follow.
3. Lean ham or cold chicken. One or two wholemeal crispbread and *Flora*. Half grapefruit to follow.
4. Cottage cheese, baked jacket potato. Half grapefruit to follow.

Numbers 3 and 4 should not be taken jointly more than three days per week (ie, 2×No 3 and 1×No 4 or 1×No 3 and 2×No 4). Neither should be taken three times.

Evening meal — select from:
1. Lean meat or poultry with two fresh green and one root vegetable. Fresh fruit other than bananas to follow.
2. Any vegetarian savoury, excluding dairy produce, with baked jacket potato and one fresh green and one fresh root vegetable. Melon, grapes, or stewed apple to follow.
3. Brown rice, brown pasta or pulses with fresh vegetables to choice (including peppers, etc) Small side salad. Half grapefruit to follow.
4. Brown rice with chicken and vegetable dish. Melon or grapes to follow.
5. Fish (not fried) with three fresh vegetables. Grapes, stewed apple or melon to follow.

Numbers 1 and 4 should not be taken more than three times per week jointly and never on the same day as lunch No 3.

Drinks

encouraged	occasionally	very rarely
dandelion	China tea	red wine
coffee	with lemon	brandy
grapefruit	decaffeinated	vodka
juice	coffee	Indian tea
mineral and	white wine	coffee
spring	*Campari*	
water	beer	
apple juice		
herbal teas		
Postum		
Barley Cup		
(Instant cereal		
beverage)		

It will be seen from the above diet that dairy produce and animal fats are kept to a low level, and that fresh vegetables, salads and fruits form a significant part of the dietary intake. The size of each meal should be dictated by appetite, as our needs vary not only from person to person but from day to day, dependent on the amount of activity undertaken and our own mental state. Eating between meals causes the digestive system to keep coming into action and thus wastes energy and reduces elimination. Anyone finding themselves hungry between meals should just increase the amount eaten at each meal, keeping the balance of contents the same throughout. When the appetite is small, a little of each constituent part of each meal should be taken, rather than one part in isolation.

A period of some two to three months on a balanced diet is necessary for the body to begin to create a healthy state of function, particularly if a less balanced diet has been followed for a long time. Once a noticeable improvement has been achieved and the general level of fitness has risen in association with some steady physical activity, it is then necessary to consider whether one's body is properly proportioned in relation to the sport which is being undertaken. Where bulk and increased muscle power are required, these can be achieved by correct use of diet in relation to concentrated training and by the use of weights and intensive repetition exercise.

In competitive sport nowadays, there is a great tendency for drugs, particularly anabolic steroids, to be used as a rapid means of producing muscle development and body bulk. The danger of this as a means of achieving an end cannot be exaggerated, and it is pleasing that there is a huge world-wide movement to ban and detect the use of drugs used as a means of improving one's sporting performance. The correct manner of producing the required body state may take a little longer but, instead of decreasing the body's health in the long term, it improves it.

What follows is an effective two-month programme for building body bulk, but this diet must *only* be used in relation to heavily increased physical activity of a specific muscle and body-building nature. It should *not* be followed for day-to-day use with normal sporting activities.

First Month

Breakfast

First day: Two poached eggs on two slices of wholewheat toast, followed by a cup of *Complan* with a mashed banana.

Second day: Muesli with grated raw apple, softened with apple juice and soaked or simmered raisins followed by two lightly boiled eggs with wholemeal toast.

Lunch

Every day: Large varied raw salad with soya protein. One large or two small baked jacket potatoes and cottage cheese, followed by mashed banana with cup of *Complan.*

Evening meal

First day: Chicken, fish or lean meat (not fried) with baked jacket potato and two fresh vegetables. Muesli and yogurt to follow.

Second day: Any vegetarian savoury with baked jacket potato, carrots and one other vegetable. Yogurt, grapes, and stewed apple to follow.

Drinks

Mid-morning and on retiring — *Complan*. Otherwise, any fresh fruit juice or dandelion coffee when thirsty between meals. Do not drink with meals other than when indicated.

Second Month

Breakfast

First day: Muesli with grated raw apple and soaked or simmered raisins, followed by two slices of wholewheat toast with baked beans and grilled tomatoes.

Second day: Three slices of wholewheat toast with grated raw carrot, followed by *Complan* with one or two mashed bananas.

Lunch

Every day: Large varied raw salad with nuts, nutmeat or soya protein. One or two baked jacket potatoes with cottage cheese followed by mashed banana with cup of *Biobalm*.

Evening meal

First day: Chicken, fish or lean meat (not fried) with baked jacket potato and at least two fresh vegetables. Muesli with grated raw apple, chopped banana and yogurt sprinkled with wheatgerm.

Second day: Any vegetarian savoury with baked jacket potato, carrots, parsnips and one green vegetable. Yogurt with mashed banana. Stewed apple and raisins to follow.

Drinks

Three times daily, *Complan*, otherwise any fresh fruit juice or dandelion coffee when thirsty between meals. Do not drink with meals other than when indicated.

After the two-month period, the normal diet (listed earlier) should be returned to but consistent exercise should be maintained. If further bulk is required, then the diets for the first and second months of the body-building plan should be used for two weeks each and the day-to-day diet followed for one month in repetition. By following this programme, weight can steadily be built up, muscle bulk can be increased, and no damage is being done to the body's ability to function. What follows is a simple list of 'do's' and 'don'ts' in relation to eating:

Do:

— eat regularly at regular times.
— drink between meals.
— drink sufficient to quench thirst only.
— eat food in its natural or as near natural state as possible.
— eat in a relaxed frame of mind.
— be guided by appetite on quantity.

Don't

— vary times of eating.
— eat between meals.
— drink with meals.
— rush or gobble meals.
— over-eat.
— eat white flour, white sugar and highly processed foods.

Drinking is also an important part of maintaining health and, as can be seen from the diets, this should be controlled as much as eating. Alcohol is obviously not a great help in relation to maintaining health and fitness, and the more serious the approach to sport, the more important it is to limit the intake of alcohol to a minimum. Where alcohol is consumed, it is better taken in the form of beer or wine, rather than spirits and mixers, and if the wine is diluted with a natural spring or mineral water, then this also helps the body to process the alcoholic input.

It is difficult to over-emphasize the importance of diet in relation to an individual's ability to compete successfully in a sporting world. There is a great advantage to be gained by improving one's dietary habits and, therefore, bodily state for sport, because in the process one's general health for everyday life will improve dramatically.

KEEPING YOUR BODY IN TRIM

In order to undertake or compete successfully in any physical activity, the body must be able to move as freely as our individual shape and size allows, and have no undue restrictions caused by bad posture or body usage in everyday life.

The key to a mobile and active body is the state of the spine, since this controls, to a very large extent, the function of the rest of the body. Abnormal spinal state has a major effect on the nervous system which is the body's telegraph system relaying messages from muscles and other tissues to and from the brain.

Exercise routine to maintain spinal mobility
The following exercises are illustrated in the Centre Section.

(Exercise 37)
Cat Stretch — commence with 10, build up to 20.
(Exercise 38)
Forehead to knee — commence with 5, build up to 15.
(Exercise 39)
Opposite arm and leg stretch — commence with 5, build up to 15.
(Exercise 3)
Trunk twisting — commence with 5, build up to 10.
(Exercise 1)
Hip rotation — commence with 5, build up to 10.
(Exercise 2)
Side stretching — commence with 5, build up to 15.

(Exercise 4)
Hands between legs — commence with 5, build up to 20.
(Exercise 49)
Abdominal press — commence with 10, build up to 20.
(Exercise 50)
Chest raises — commence with 5, build up to 20.
(Exercise 51)
Leg lifts — commence with 5, build up to 20.
(Exercise 52)
Salmon raise — commence with 5, build up to 20.
(Exercise 43)
Kneeling press ups — commence with 10, build up to 15.
(Exercise 53)
Alternate knee raises — commence with 5, build up to 15.
(Exercise 40)
Sit-ups to alternate knees — commence with 5, build up to 15.
(Exercise 41)
Sit-ups to both knees — commence with 5, build up to 10.
(Exercise 23)
Arm swinging — commence with 10 each side, build up to 15.
(Exercise 5)
Jogging and running on the spot — commence to a count of 10 and work up to a count of 30 for each phase (described but not illustrated in Centre Section).

As can be seen from the diagram, in normality there is a gentle 's' curve to the

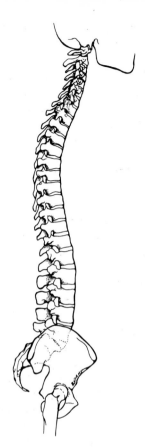

Normal
spine

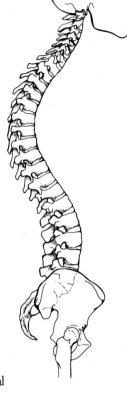

Abnormal
spine

spine in which position the pelvis is properly aligned and the legs, which are attached to the pelvis at the hip joints, are able to move through a normal plane. In this position, the balancing muscle structures at the front and the back of the body and legs are the normal length and power in relation to each other. At the upper end of the spine, the shoulders will be maintained in a correct position which means that the chest can function normally during breathing and that the arms have a normal range of movement. The muscles of the chest and back will also be in balanced and harmonic relationship.

If the curvature of the spine is disturbed then this balanced relationship between opposing muscle groups disappears: certain groups become shortened and others will be lengthened, dependent upon which way the pelvis and the shoulders have moved. Equally, if the pelvis is tilted forward, then this will be compensated for at the upper end of the spine by an opposite movement of the shoulders and vice versa. When the pelvis tilts forward, the muscles on the front of the thigh become stretched, with appropriate compensation up the whole length of the spine and a gradual onset of a compensating spinal curvature. Whilst this may not cause many visible problems for some years in day-to-day life, if one suddenly introduces strenuous activity, then these are the areas which can be highly vulnerable to traumatic damage under running, turning and twisting conditions. One only has to look at the shapes of various people playing sport, especially at amateur and surprisingly frequently at professional levels, to appreciate that potential injury sources exist which are nothing to do with the sport itself.

In order to be an effective competitor in sport, one must be aware of the body in one's normal day-to-day situations, and attempt to maintain it in the best possible state to enable us to compete effectively in our chosen leisure activity. Since gravity is constantly squashing us (which is fairly fortunate, since otherwise we would tend to float off the face of the earth) we have to try to offset its effects with a conscious effort to lengthen and elongate the spine. The old maxim of 'stand tall, walk tall, sit tall' should be remembered at all times, and we should try to visualize ourselves stretching out from the head down rather than pressing down on to the feet. If one hangs a pair of trousers on a hanger by the waistband then, when the bottom of the trousers is resting on the ground, they will be crumpled and creased. As the hanger is raised, they will gradually fall into shape and, as the trousers clear the ground, all the creases will disappear. We should visualize our body in this fashion and try to see ourselves taking all the 'creases' out of the body by lifting the head and neck to offset the gravitational pressure.

It is important with postural training not to adopt a posture in a military fashion which is rigid, stiff and immobile. Posture is in reality a state of bodily awareness in which as few muscles as possible are being used to maintain a normal position, maximum mobility is available at any given moment,

and alignment of the body and the position of the body's centre of gravity is as near correct as possible. This sounds complicated initially, but, when analysed, is not too difficult so long as one creates the interest to become aware of what one is doing with the body at all times.

The alignment factor is very critical since the point at which the body's weight is directed through to the earth has a major effect on feet, knees, legs and hips. If one is leaning too far forward, the centre of gravity actually falls outside the feet which means that the knees have to be locked back rather than being in a relaxed position, which is normal, and the hips are placed under constant stress. This means that movement eventually becomes restricted and joint and muscle damage is much more likely to occur. It also means that the arches of the feet are liable to collapse and that the ankles are going to be under great pressure. When the body is correctly positioned, the weight falls straight through the arch of the foot, and, as with bridge building, it is this pressure on the centre of the arch which maintains it in a normal state of function. Flat feet and fallen arches lead to many more serious problems later on if sport is undertaken without any attempt to correct what is nearly always a problem of functional posture rather than any specific hereditary abnormality. There are, of course, people who do have inherent problems and, in these cases, advice is often needed in relation to support or particular footwear which can help to relieve the otherwise detrimental effects of this abnormality.

Once we have become aware of what the body is doing, it will be seen that in most cases a lot of muscles are being used which are not necessary for day-to-day use. Sitting in a chair or a car, large groups of muscles are frequently undertaking activity which has no relationship to the movements being carried out at that particular time. If this can be noticed and controlled, two major benefits in body performance result. Firstly, the energy which is being wasted is suddenly saved, and, secondly, the muscles which would otherwise tend to become stiff, maintain a relaxed and normal tone and function. It is important to remember that no improvement will take place until we make the effort to find out where misuse is occurring.

A regular exercise programme to maintain the mobility of the spine and to keep the postural muscles in good tone should be undertaken on a daily basis. Below is a sensible programme of exercises for the average person to undertake, and this should be repeated morning and evening. The quantity can be increased once it becomes easy to carry out the whole programme, but only as far as double the quantity since, after this, no useful effect will be served. The exercises are not to build huge bulging muscles or make a sporting superstar, but to maintain a healthy spine and a full range of mobility for the major joints of the body so that any specialization of technique can be carried on from this platform.

Warm up routine suitable for any sport
The following exercises are illustrated in the Centre Section.

(Exercise 1)
Hip rotation — commence with 10, build up to 15.
(Exercise 2)
Side stretching — commence with 5, build up to 10.
(Exercise 4)
Hands between legs — commence with 5, build up to 10.

(Exercise 9)
Alternate leg stretch — commence with 5 each way, build up to 10.
(Exercise 29)
Wall stretch — leave legs up wall for a count of 30.
(Exercise 42)
Hip stretch — attempt until tired.
(Exercise 10)
Arm stretch — repeat until tired.
(Exercise 11)
Neck stretch — repeat 5 times each way.
(Exercise 5)
Jogging on the spot — commence to a count of 20, building up to 30 (described but not illustrated in Centre Section).

Warming up is a very important factor in relation to undertaking any strenuous physical exercise and one which, sadly, is in many cases almost completely ignored, particularly by the amateur. To warm up satisfactorily for any sport, the programme above should be undertaken. It is quite brief but the benefits of using it are much more far-reaching. The stretching exercises should never be forced: they should be relaxed into rather than pushed into and, as greater proficiency is reached, each exercise position may be held for a longer time.

Any sport does and will involve the possibility of injury, and these will occur from time to time. Injuries are discussed in greater detail in the final chapter, and some advice on treatment is given. However, if a healthy general physical state is achieved, regular exercise undertaken and proper warm-up procedures followed, then the liability to injury will be dramatically reduced before any form of play or activity commences.

Active fitness cannot be contemplated without considering breathing, since this is one of the most important functions the body has to undertake, particularly under stress and increased activity. The primary function of breathing is not, as many think, to take in oxygen but more importantly to eliminate carbon dioxide. Until the bloodstream is cleared of carbon dioxide, it is impossible for it to absorb oxygen and, therefore, the out-breath is the most critical. A good out-breath is always followed by an involuntary inhalation as the muscles relax so, therefore, as long as one concentrates on exhaling efficiently, then the inhalation becomes a natural part of the process. Excessive carbon dioxide in the bloodstream is a major factor in exhaustion problems, and particularly affects mental concentration.

It must be remembered that the lungs are pear-shaped, with the widest part at the base of the chest, and that the diaphragm, the muscle responsible for a large proportion of the breathing activity, is also across the base of the chest cavity. The lungs can be considered to function like a pair of bellows — ie, to breathe in, the base of the chest has to be opened, and to breathe out it has to be closed. This means that on breathing in, the upper part of the abdomen and the diaphragm should expand and the chest wall enlarge sideways: on breathing out it should collapse, with the abdomen flattening completely, to help push the unwanted air out of the lung cavities. This is the absolute opposite to the traditional military breath —

ie, breathing in with the top of the chest expanding and pulling the stomach flat, and everything collapsing on the outward breath. If increased activity is to be undertaken, to learn to breathe correctly is absolutely fundamental to the body's ability to function efficiently.

As physical activity increases, the need for oxygen intake and carbon dioxide output also increases, and so it is important to know how to step up this function. The first manner is always to increase the size of the breath and not the rate of breathing, as this is a much more effective and efficient way of the exchange taking place. Therefore, the more energy one uses and the more activity one undertakes, the deeper the breathing must become. Panting should only take place in conditions of extreme stress when, in fact, the body has gone on to self control because of the demands that have been made upon it.

The whole cardiovascular system is affected by the correct breathing action — the diaphragm acts as a large massaging unit and stimulates heart function. At the same time the abdominal muscle quality is improved because the same action increases the tension of the abdominal muscle wall and this, in its turn, helps to support the lower back. Thus, correct breathing not only helps improve fitness from the air-exchange point of view but it is also an integral part of the maintenance of proper body function.

GETTING FIT FOR GENERAL SPORTS

Once any person intending to undertake sport as a means of constructively filling leisure time has come to grips with the need for the personal effort required to raise one's fitness to a suitable level, then the basis is laid for trouble-free enjoyment. In the previous chapters, general fitness and awareness have been discussed, and unless attention is paid to these factors any efforts to indulge in sport will almost certainly have some long or short-term detrimental effect.

In later chapters, a large number of sports will be discussed individually, and particular problems of each looked at with a view to helping to avoid injuries, strains and limitations to fitness, whilst achieving the best possible level of competitiveness. This book is not, nor is it meant to be, a coaching manual for each sport, but it is intended to provide guidance as to how to reach a suitable platform on which skilled coaches can develop individual techniques in particular sports.

In most sports and athletics, coaching has become very technical and the results achieved by competitors throughout the world are startling in their rapid improvement. The problem which goes hand in hand with this development is that many athletes and sports persons are suffering more long and short-term injuries. The main reason for this is that coaching has been based so carefully on the individual sport or skill that general fitness mobility and overall body balance have frequently been overlooked. By learning sensible dietary control, becoming aware of how the body is used, taking adequate regular exercise and practising mobility routines, then it becomes possible to reach the maximum viable level in whatever sport the individual pursues, without side effects, which also means that one can generally improve further still.

The more involved one is in sport, and the more professional in terms of the need to win, the more important it is to realize that sport is a seven days a week undertaking. One or two coaching sessions a week and playing or competing in the sport at the weekend is not the complete way to achieve full satisfaction competitively, or to maintain an improved fitness. Everything one does in the way of sitting, standing, moving, eating, drinking, and relaxing generally should be done with physical fitness in mind.

There are many forms of 'keep fit classes', gymnasiums, weight training rooms, aerobic studios and dancing classes. All these activities have their merits, but many of them are run by people untrained or only partly trained in the particular skill, and in these cases a little knowledge can be a dangerous thing. Many people have ended on the physiotherapist's couch or the osteopath's table because of injuries sustained undertaking either excessive exercise too quickly, or movements unsuited to the particular individual. If classes of this sort are to be attended, it is still important to be fit to start with and, above all, to make certain that the instructor in charge of the class has an adequate training in that particular skill. An instructor should also be notified of any particular problems which may have been suffered by the individual up to that point. It is no good going to an aerobics class having had backache for many months, not telling the instructor, and then being surprised when acute pain follows.

Weight training is increasingly popular and, carefully controlled in the right circumstances, it can produce considerable increases in body size and fitness. Generally speaking, weight machines where the back is supported throughout, are infinitely less dangerous than using simple weight bars. It is very easy to move a fraction out of alignment while lifting a weight in an unsupported position, and dramatically change the area of pressure in the spine, thus causing damage. Unless the preparation and instruction in the use of weights is very skilled, it is much better to use static machines, particularly *Nautilus*, which have the ability to develop specific muscles without potential spinal damage. Even these machines, if badly or excessively used, can cause damage, so the maxim is 'softly, softly, catchee monkey'.

The use of weights as an integrated part of a fitness programme to prepare for another sport can be very beneficial, and their sensible control can produce muscle development of benefit to whatever particular activity is to be undertaken, but again the coach of the specific activity should be aware of what is being done in the course of preparation. Any physical activity other than the basic fitness programmes outlined in this book may conflict with the particular areas which coaches in individual sports wish to develop.

Weight lifting as a sport in its own right is becoming increasingly popular, and all the guidelines mentioned must be applied with some discipline if damage is not to ensue. The low back, knees and legs are particularly prone to problems and, therefore, low back mobility exercises should always be used prior to and post lifting.

The exercise programme laid out in 'Keeping your body in trim' should be used morning and evening and within a half-hour before and after practising or competing. Advice on supportive belts should always be taken, and it is much better to be safe than sorry if in doubt about a particular lift. Because of the static nature of the sport, it is also important to make sure that mobility is not lost in the legs, hips and knees, and these should be regularly used for other forms of exercise, particularly swimming, to maintain the necessary mobility to prevent rheumatic and arthritic problems in later life.

Field events are another area where great physical strength is a prime requirement of the sport, and once again a seven-day commitment to increasing fitness is totally necessary if strains and damages are not to occur. It is another area where good coaching is essential and anyone interested in competing in these events should always make sure that sound advice is available.

British sports such as rounders, stool ball, skittles, bowling, ten-pin bowling, etc, all involve physical activity to a greater or lesser degree, and should be viewed with sufficient seriousness to undertake the simple mobility and fitness exercises previously recommended. Running or some other aerobic activity should be undertaken in preparation for the more energetic of those sports, while walking can provide suitable preparation for the more leisurely activities such as bowls. A lot of bending and stretching goes on in the course of a few ends of bowls and, unless the player is prepared, it can have painful results.

For obvious reasons, not every sport can be dealt with in depth, but an effort has been made to deal with the bulk of those undertaken in large numbers. For those competing in sports which are not played in Britain, the training programme used should be that of the sport most akin to the particular national game. For example, American Football and Australian Rules have very similar physical requirements to rugby, and, if the rugby training advice is used as a basis for competitors in these sports, then they will have achieved a physical starting point for development into their own game.

In the following chapters, sports are looked at individually with a view to helping the budding competitor avoid the pitfalls and enjoy the pleasures of his or her chosen area of involvement.

1. RUNNING, JOGGING AND ATHLETICS

Athletics, jogging and running, particularly marathon running, are activities with greatly increasing numbers of enthusiastic followers. One only has to look at the response to fundraising mini-marathons and full marathons to see the number of people who are now involved in this form of exercise.

There has been a great boom in jogging but, sad to say, many people have suffered injuries, discomfort and long-term problems through undertaking jogging inadequately equipped or prepared. The first vitally important step to ensure the minimum of problems is to purchase the correct footwear. Despite warnings otherwise, many people still jog in ordinary trainers or flat-soled tennis shoes or similar. The effect of jogging in these is to cause a lot of shock to the spine, often with resultant backache or pain. In poor footwear also lies the potential for damage to the leg muscles, with the very frequent occurrence of a condition called 'shin splints' — characterized by pain on the front of the shin, with any effort to come up on the toes causing extreme discomfort.

Proper jogging/running shoes should be worn with an elevated heel and preferably of the air sole variety as this cushions any shock to the spine even further. It is a totally false economy to buy a cheap pair of shoes when they are such an important item. One should also make sure that they fit comfortably and well, and that the heel tag of the shoe does not put too much pressure on the Achilles tendon at the back of the heel. Excessive pressure on this tendon just above the bony part of the heel can cause either inflammation and soreness of the tendon itself, or, in some cases, permanent damage to the fibres of the tendon. If any pain is experienced in any of the above areas, it is sensible to get professional advice to find the cause of the problem, and to undertake prompt remedial action.

Jogging, as such, is not necessarily the boost to physical improvement that many people think. Because of the unstressed nature of the sport, the available cardiovascular improvement can be obtained within a few weeks. It is far more effective to run rather than jog, to spend a little more time up on the toes rather than purely flat on the heel, and to push oneself steadily a little harder to achieve a continuing improvement in cardiovascular function. A shorter but more energetic run is generally more effective physically than a slow and steady long jog.

For jogging, running or athletics, it is important to warm up prior to going out, even for a steady jog. Presuming one has undertaken the regular daily exercises discussed in 'Keeping your body in trim', all that is necessary for jogging or running is adequate stretching and then a steady start to activity, building up to desired speed in a short space of time. The stretching exercises given here loosen the appropriate muscles in the body and help considerably to prevent any pulls or tears during the course of the activity. It is surprising, even with comparatively gentle jogging, how much damage one can do by failing to stretch off before undertaking the activity.

Stretching exercises
(Illustrated in Centre Section)

(Exercise 37)
Cat Stretch — commence with 10, build up
  to 20.
(Exercise 38)
Forehead to knee — commence with 5, build
  up to 15.
(Exercise 2)
Side stretching — commence with 5 each
  way, build up to 10.
(Exercise 1)
Hip rotation — do 10 each way.
(Exercise 3)
Trunk twisting — do 10 each way.
(Exercise 39)
Opposite arm and leg stretch — commence
  with 5, build up to 15.

For specific athletics and more competitive running, it is even more important that adequate warming up and stretching is undertaken and this should be specifically related to whichever event one is about to participate in. All good coaches can advise on a suitable routine for one particular sport and this advice should always be sought and followed.

After running, jogging or any sport, it is essential to 'warm down' rather than cease activity suddenly. One should always slow down gently at the end of a run so that one reduces heart function gradually and then walk around while the body cools down to a more normal temperature. One of the most damaging things to do is to stop suddenly when hot and sit down without letting the body cool off first. This produces stiffness and tightness in the muscles and can build up problems for the next time any activity is undertaken. Once the body has cooled down adequately, it should always be washed or showered, preferably the latter, at a temperature only just above blood heat. After washing and adequate all-over exposure to the water, a brief cold shower will stimulate skin tone and improve peripheral circulation. This cold shower should not be taken until adequately cooled down by the earlier procedures — then it is most effective.

Injuries may be sustained by tripping, or twisting one's ankle whilst running, particularly on cross-country routes or on uneven surfaces, and advice on remedial treatment of these sorts of injuries is available further on in the book. One should always try to select one's routes for jogging or running with care — the more time spent on soft ground the less the chance of any damage to spine or legs. Equally, the more time spent on uneven ground the greater the potential of damage to the joints, owing to tripping or falling.

For those competitors involved in short and highly explosive running, ie, sprinting or even upper-class middle-distance running, the dangers of muscle damage are very much higher. The more explosive the action, the greater the probability of strains and tears becomes. For these athletes, adequate stretching and warming up is absolutely vital and should *never* be ignored.

Whilst training for track events, one of the major causes of long-term problems, particularly with ham-string injuries, is running around tracks perpetually in an anti-clockwise direction. Because all races are run in this direction, it is habitual for training to be done in the same fashion. Consistently pushing off one leg when entering a bend — ie, the right leg with anti-clockwise running — gradually causes an imbalance at the pelvic level and the athlete ends with one leg effectively shorter than the other. This causes a tendency to ham-string strain and damage, and has affected many top athletes, including those of Olympic gold medal calibre like Sebastian Coe.

Apart from normal background training and running when doing track training, the way to avoid the lop-sided problem is to do at least thirty per cent of the training running in the opposite direction. By covering a reasonable distance, pushing hard in the opposite direction, the body is able to compensate for the uneven stresses and this avoids many potential areas of lasting injury.

Athletics, running and jogging are, in theory, some of the safest ways of taking competitive exercise. They only become a problem to the enthusiast if adequate preparation is not done, if training regimes are not carefully pursued, and if good coaching is not available. The latter is very important in events where technique is critical, as even careful preparation can be worthless if one is not taught how to execute the particular skills in an efficient way. Those interested in athletics should always make the effort to join a good club with good coaching facilities where their potential can be fulfilled.

2. TENNIS

Modern day tennis is a very much harder and faster game than it was a few years ago, with the result that there are far more injuries sustained playing tennis than was previously the case. At a professional level, the speed of the game, the number of games played and the travelling involved from match to match have produced a group of very fine players, nearly all of whom at some stage or other in their careers have had injury problems.

Because of the sheer physical strength required to consistently hit the ball hard, and because of the amount of body mobility required to produce and to counteract heavy spin, the low back is particularly vulnerable and one only has to look at sports pages in papers to see the number of top professionals missing games because of back injuries. Many of these injuries are the result of failure in the early playing years to maintain the back's mobility whilst training and playing for many hours.

Tennis is very much a one-sided game — if you look at most senior professionals, one side of their body is twenty or thirty per cent larger than the other side. Because of this uneven muscle pull, spinal curvature is a real danger. Once a curvature begins to develop, then the back is vulnerable to any awkward movement, slip, fall or strain, as the body's normal safety margin has already gone. So often, although the injury may appear to have happened on the spot, it is the poor training in the years preceding the one particular movement that really made the injury a reality.

For both amateurs and professionals it is vital that adequate warming up is done before playing, and that a good series of stretching exercises are undertaken. Presuming one uses a morning loosening programme already, a sensible and effective loosening and stretching routine to be used prior to any practice or playing of tennis is given here. If proper preparation is not done, whilst no injury may be felt at the time, long-term damage is being stored up to produce problems at the least convenient time as far as the sport is concerned.

Loosening and stretching routine
(Illustrated in Centre Section)

(Exercise 37)
Cat stretch — commence with 10, build up to 20.
(Exercise 1)
Hip rotation — do 5 each way.
(Exercise 2)
Side stretching — commence with 5, build up to 10.
(Exercise 12)
Shoulder shrugs — repeat between 5 and 10 times each way.
(Exercise 9)
Alternate leg stretch — commence with 5, build up to 10.
(Exercise 44)
Sitting leg stretch — commence with 5, build up to 15.
(Exercise 42)
Hip stretch — do 5 each side.
(Exercise 4)
Hands between legs — repeat 10 times.
(Exercise 6)
Jog and hop — continue until a reasonable

degree of cardiovascular stimulation is achieved (described but not illustrated in Centre Section).

If more than one match is to be played in the course of a day, then the routine should be repeated before the start of each game. One should also be very careful between matches to make sure that suitable outer clothing is worn in order to keep the body temperature fairly even, and that no sudden chilling takes place. It is important to keep moving around until body temperature has returned to normal, after which one may relax without fear of stiffening up. After the final game, the warming down process is even more important and one should make sure that one does not shower until one has cooled down, and the shower should be of not much above blood heat, followed by a short, sharp cold shower to stimulate the peripheral circulation.

To counteract the dangers of the one-sidedness of the game, it is important to develop the opposite side of the body to the side used to play, and also to make sure that during all two-sided exercises the same amount of movement and rotation is achieved on both sides of the body. If there is any tendency for one side to be more mobile than the other, one should work on the less mobile side until the movement evens out.

Exercises to ensure even-sided muscle development (Illustrated in Centre Section)

(Exercise 13)
Arm flex with weight — continue until muscle begins to feel fatigue.
(Exercise 14)
Arm exercise using weight — continue until tired.

(Exercise 15)
Contra-pressure exercise — continue until some degree of muscle fatigue is felt.
(Exercise 18)
One arm push — commence with 5, build up to 20.
(Exercise 19)
Wall push and rotate — continue until tired.
(Exercise 17)
Racquet swing — continue until tired.

The series of exercises outlined here can be used either left or right sided, dependent on which hand one plays with, to level out development of the main muscles used in the course of tennis. So long as balance is maintained, not only will the spine remain in the correct alignment but actual body balance will be improved and, therefore, the ability to use one's expertise to the full is increased.

Problems with the shoulders and particularly with the elbow have interfered with many amateurs' and professionals' playing careers, and should always be correctly dealt with. Tennis elbow is very common, and is usually caused either by a miss-hit ball or, more frequently, by playing with a racquet with too small a grip. There is a great tendency for people to use a small-handled racquet which appears to give more confidence, but which greatly increases the strain on the wrist and elbow joint in particular.

If serious pain develops the joint should be rested, and alternate hot and cold bathing is a very effective means of treating the site of the pain. This consists of two bowls of water, one as hot as is comfortably bearable, and the other as cold as it runs from the tap. The elbow should be placed in the hot for three minutes, the cold for one minute, and the process then repeated, so that the total treatment time is eight minutes. This should be repeated two or three times during the course of the day. The process may also be aided by placing a handful of Epsom salts into the hot water prior to immersion. If the elbow or shoulder fails to respond to rest and water treatment, then it is important that a suitably qualified sports injury specialist should be consulted, because the more serious cases, if neglected, can be very long and painful injuries.

The varying surfaces of tennis courts can all have an effect on players, and once again proper equipment comes into play. Nowadays, there are sophisticated designs of tennis shoe sole which make a huge difference to the ability to maintain good footing on surfaces as different as clay, artificial grass, and real grass. So long as finance permits, it is preferable to make sure that the risk of slips and falls is reduced by wearing the correct footwear, than to suffer the alternative. The court surface dramatic-ally affects the pace of the game, and particularly when playing on grass the value of being well warmed up, stretched and loose before the game is even greater. The more tennis that is played on hard surfaces, the more important good footwear becomes as there is undoubtedly greater stress on the legs and low back in these conditions.

As with most sports, it is always easier to play the game correctly, and good coaching at an early stage is bound to reduce the number of injuries caused by miss-hitting and miss-timing the ball. It should be remembered that the ball is travelling at a considerable rate and, therefore, the shock involved at the moment of impact is quite great. There is no doubt that modern tennis racquets are much better designed to absorb the impact of the ball, and for anybody who has tendency to wrist or elbow problems, large or mid-sized racquets can be very helpful in preventing further or recurring injury.

3. SQUASH

Squash is a very popular sport today, partly because it offers scope for physically energetic exercise irrespective of the weather, and in not too long a period of time. Unlike team games or games such as golf, one does not need three or four hours to have a game of squash. It is this very convenience that is one of the greatest potential dangers of the sport.

Many people who play squash lead very sedentary lives, and tend to follow a life-style which is not conducive to general physical well-being. To play once or twice a week without any other strenuous exercise and, in most cases, without even warming up or stretching initially, is not only liable to cause all sorts of muscular and joint problems but, more importantly, can have a very detrimental effect on the heart and the cardiovascular system. Being a physically intensive sport, squash is one which requires a high level of fitness if the player is to be able to continue to play on a regular basis without creating both short and long-term health problems.

To be able to play without worrying, one must take exercise on a regular basis, over and above the general daily exercises recommended earlier. Running at least twice a week for a minimum of fifteen minutes, preferably twenty, should be a regular part of the squash player's training programme. The run should start off with five minutes jogging, then five minutes of short sprints, followed by steady running, followed by short sprints, followed by steady running, etc. This should be followed by five minutes medium pace running with a slow tail-down towards the end of the run so that, by the time one returns to base, breathing and pulse have steadied down considerably. At the end of this run, one should walk around until normal body temperature and pulse have been regained. Intersperse this period with stretching and mobility exercises. Stretching exercises should also be practised for a few minutes each evening, because the nature of the game demands that muscles perform considerable feats of stretching and position change: therefore, mobility and elasticity are essential to preventing injury in the muscular system.

Warming up and stretching exercises
(Illustrated in Centre Section)
(Exercise 1)
Hip rotation — repeat 5 times each way.
(Exercise 3)
Trunk twisting — repeat 5 times each way.
(Exercise 2)
Side stretching — commence with 5, build up to 10.
(Exercise 4)
Hands between legs — repeat 10 times.
(Exercise 9)
Alternate leg stretch — repeat 5 times each way.
(Exercise 44)
Sitting leg stretch — repeat 5 times each way.
(Exercise 45)
Touching alternate feet — repeat 10 times each way.
(Exercise 5)
Jogging on the spot — repeat until a degree of muscular warmth is achieved (described but not illustrated in Centre Section).

Before starting any game, a proper warming up and stretching routine should be undertaken, and a similar routine should be followed after the game, whilst allowing the body to settle down without creating stiffness and tension. Once the routine is over, then a warm shower should be taken, followed, where possible, by a short cold one. One should ensure that after a game of squash one does not get physically cold and suitable clothing should be worn as necessary.

To prevent ankle injuries, one must make sure that proper shoes are worn for squash. Apart from preserving the surface of the court, they are designed to give adequate support to the ankle which is necessary because of the turning and twisting which takes place. Ill-fitting squash shoes or shoes which are not really squash shoes have caused many foot and ankle injuries which can be very painful and cause the player to miss some weeks of squash until the pain subsides.

It is also necessary to make sure that the size of the grip of the racquet is correct, or problems may be experienced with the wrist and forearm. Elbow problems are much less prevalent in squash than in tennis, because the manner of hitting the ball and the amount of power used is much less conducive to elbow damage. The wrist, however, suffers considerable strain and any player should ensure that wrists are strengthened and mobile if the game is to be played well and without difficulties. Either a wrist exerciser or an old tennis ball which can be squeezed between the fingers are very good tools for building up the strength of the wrist and forearm. This should be done with both hands, otherwise uneven bodily development can result.

To avoid any spinal problems because of the one-sided nature of the game, one should follow daily the brief exercise programme laid out below which should be done with whichever is the non-striking side.

Exercises to maintain even-sided muscle development (Illustrated in Centre Section)

(Exercise 19)
Wall push and rotate — commence with 5, build up to 15.
(Exercise 14)
Arm exercise using weight — repeat until the arm feels tired.
(Exercise 18)
One arm push — repeat the muscle feels tired.
(Exercise 54)
One-handed press up — attempt 5.
(Exercise 15)
Contra-pressure exercise 1 — repeat until the muscle feels tired.
(Exercise 16)
Contra-pressure exercise 2 — continue until the muscle feels warm.

If this advice is followed, then it is quite possible to play squash to 'a ripe old age' and for it to be of great benefit in the maintenance of physical and mental fitness and well-being. However, if not sensibly approached, it is a game that can result in long-term problems which can totally affect future health.

4. BADMINTON

Because of the far greater number of halls and sports centres available for playing the sport over the last few years, badminton has become even more popular as a recreational activity. It is a game which spans a broad age bracket, and which in fact is far more energetic and tiring than it may appear to be initially.

A good basic level of fitness is required to play the game successfully, and the advice given in the initial chapters of the book should be followed to improve the general level of the body's function. The game requires short, explosive bursts of activity, and good hand-eye co-ordination and reflex speed. These are only obtainable if good preparation work has been done prior to commencing play.

To increase stamina and to improve general cardiovascular fitness, at least two runs a week should be used as part of the basic fitness programme — each of about twenty minutes duration. This should consist of five minutes jogging, ten minutes running and five minutes jogging, after which the back mobility exercises shown below should be done until heart rate returns to nearly normal. This should then be followed by a body-heat shower and, where available, a short, sharp, cold shower before changing.

Warming up before a game is very important, since a large number of the injuries suffered by badminton players are muscle pulls and strains which occur because they have not been sufficiently stretched and loosened prior to the game commencing. The routine outlined below should be used preceding the game, and also after the game to make sure that no tensions or stresses are taken forward to the next period of play.

Warming up routine
(Illustrated in Centre Section)

(Exercise 37)
Cat stretch — commence with 5, build up to 20.
(Exercise 9)
Alternate leg stretch — repeat 5 times each way.
(Exercise 44)
Sitting leg stretch — repeat 5 times each way.
(Exercise 1)
Hip rotation — repeat 8 times each way.
(Exercise 3)
Trunk twisting — repeat 8 times each way.
(Exercise 46)
Knee clasp — commence with 5 to each knee, build up to 10.
(Exercise 49)
Abdominal press — repeat 10 times.
(Exercise 4)
Hands between legs — repeat 10 times.
(Exercise 29)
Wall stretch — hold for a count of 30.
(Exercise 40)
Sit-ups to alternate knees — commence with 10, build up to 20.
(Exercise 37)
Cat stretch — repeat 10 times.
(Exercise 38)
Forehead to knee — commence with 5, build up to 20.

If a number of games are being played, it is important to make sure that one keeps warm between the games, and if the interval is more than a few minutes, then a short series of the above exercises should again be used prior to playing.

Although badminton is a one-sided sport, the relatively light weight of the racquet and the very mobile nature of the game to a very large extent compensate for this. Badminton players get very few major 'one-sided' problems, unlike tennis players with whom it can be a major factor. It is, however, a good idea to make sure that the left shoulder (in a right-handed player) does not suffer from a relative lack of mobility in usage, and the exercise programme set out below can make sure that this does not happen.

Exercise routine to maintain even-sided muscle development
(Illustrated in Centre Section)

(Exercise 19)
Wall push and rotate — repeat at least 10 times, build up as strength increases.

(Exercise 18)
One arm push — repeat at least 5 times.
(Exercise 22)
Arm swing — repeat at least 6 times.
(Exercise 15)
Contra-pressure exercise 1 — repeat until the muscle feels tired.

Ankles are an area of the body that can suffer problems in badminton, unless careful attention is paid to the choice of footwear. It is amazing how many people will play in sloppily fitting shoes and wonder why twisted and sprained ankles result.

The importance of being fit for badminton cannot be emphasized too much, as it tends to be played, rather like squash, by large numbers of people who do little or no exercise for most of the week and then have a fairly high intensity of activity for a short period of time. This is dangerous both from a cardiovascular point of view and also from a muscular and structural perspective.

5. CRICKET

Like most sports nowadays, even the gentlemanly art of cricket has become far more involved with physical fitness than used to be the case. Fielding has become a much more important role in the game, and athleticism is necessary in order to field at the now expected standards. Quality of equipment has improved, and this too accelerates the pace of the game to some degree.

Amateur players, who play mainly at weekends or the occasional midweek game, should never underestimate how important it is to prepare for the game during the preceding days. Cricket is a game which involves a lot of bending, crouching, turning and stopping, and, hopefully of course, running a number of times to and fro whilst encumbered with a large amount of protective padding. If adequate preparation is not made, then backaches, muscle strains and ankle and knee problems are very common.

As well as the daily routine of exercise recommended in 'Keeping your body in trim' all players should try to get at least two fifteen minute runs per week as part of a regular routine, starting off with a gentle jog and gradually building up to medium pace running after about five minutes, this being interspersed with short sprints, and for the last five minutes slowing the pace down until reasonably cooled off by return to base. Whilst the remainder of the cooling down of the body takes place, the stretching exercises outlined here should be practised to help with nimbleness and mobility in the field.

Exercise to aid mobility
(Illustrated in Centre Section)

(Exercise 4)
Hands between legs — repeat 10 times.
(Exercise 1)
Hip rotation — repeat 5 times each way.
(Exercise 2)
Side stretching — repeat 10 times each way.
(Exercise 45)
Touching alternate feet — repeat 10 times each way.
(Exercise 56)
Squatting — repeat 5 times.
(Exercise 20)
Squatting star jumps — commence with 8, work up to 20.

For serious batsmen and particularly for the wicket keeper, a very good warm-up training is to exercise and do some running wearing an old pair of pads. To do a series of squats, squat thrusts, and shuttle runs whilst strapped into the pads helps to muscle up the legs for the more difficult art of running and moving whilst thus encumbered.

Another problem frequently suffered by batsmen is stiffness of the neck and shoulders. Cricket being a sideways-on game means that, in the course of a long innings, a batsman is turning his head consistently to one side for a long period of time. It is important to make sure that the neck stays mobile during everyday life, and the second set of exercises are a simple series designed to improve neck and shoulder mobility. These should be used regularly, whenever the opportunity presents itself.

Neck mobility exercises
(Illustrated in Centre Section)

(Exercise 12)
Shoulder shrugs — repeat 3 times each way.
(Exercise 11)
Neck stretch — repeat 6 times each way.
(Exercise 23)
Alternate arm swinging — repeat 5 times each side.
(Exercise 24)
Double arm swinging — repeat 5 times.

Whilst at the wicket for a long innings, doing the first four of the exercises whenever the opportunity presents itself (such as between overs or when the opposition bowler has a particularly long run!) helps not only to prevent any stiffness but also assists blood flow in the head, makes concentration better and reflex response quicker.

For bowlers, the tendency to low back injury is much greater, particularly, of course, with fast bowlers. One of the main sources of damage is when people try to bowl too fast for their own capability and subject the low back to a severe pounding in the process. Bad technique also accounts for a large number of problems as the low back is put through much excessive torsional twisting if a good, smooth sideways-on technique is not achieved. All fast bowlers need stamina and, therefore, extra running over and above the normal training programme is very sensible for anybody who wishes to take fast bowling seriously. Neck and shoulder mobility is, of course, also critical to any bowler, and the exercises for these parts should be used on a day-to-day basis to maintain as great a range of movement as is possible.

To try to minimize damage to the low back, the following exercises should be used over and above a normal daily routine for those who really wish to bowl safely at maximum pace.

Exercises to increase spinal strength and mobility (Illustrated in Centre Section)

(Exercise 37)
Cat stretch — commence with 10, build up to 20.
(Exercise 48)
Figure 'U' sit-ups — commence with 5, build up to 20.
(Exercise 57)
Leg raise 9 in, open and close — commence with 5, build up to 20.
(Exercise 52)
Salmon raise — commence with 10, build up to 20.
(Exercise 50)
Chest raise — commence with 5, build up to 20.
(Exercise 51)
Leg lifts — commence with 10, build up to 20.
(Exercise 62)
Straight leg lowering — commence with 5, build up to 15.

The object of these exercises is to increase the strength of the main postural muscles at the base of the spine, whilst maintaining the necessary mobility to make sure that damage does not occur at the moment of delivery and the subsequent follow-through. All bowlers should have a good stretch of all muscles before going onto the field, and, prior to being called to bowl, should try and warm up the whole of the body as much as is possible in the circumstances of fielding. Stretching out between balls, moving the shoulders, moving the neck, and jogging to and fro between overs all help to keep the body loose and, therefore, less vulnerable to strain.

Cricket has its own series of traumatic injuries, some of which are very painful, as anybody who has been hit on the shin by a cricket ball will vouch. There is now available a large amount of equipment which offers protection to the most vulnerable areas of the batsman's body, and also helmets for both batsmen and fielders. Whilst some players feel it is 'cissy' to wear padding and protective helmets, there have already been a number of instances where the helmets, in particular, have probably saved the life of a fielder or batsman, and there seems little point in suffering painful bruising when the correct equipment can prevent this happening. Suffering pain for its own sake is not an essential part of the game of cricket!

6. HOCKEY

Hockey is a game which has maintained a steady popularity and seems to be ever improving its standards. The results of the 1984 Olympics were a great boost for hockey in the British Isles.

The first essential for any hockey player to be competitive and to avoid any potential injuries is to make sure that adequate running stamina has been attained in training, and that a good general level of stamina has been built up. To this end, two half-hour runs per week should be taken, starting with a ten-minute steady jog or slow run, followed by ten minutes running at high pace, followed by a gradual slow-down for the last ten minutes, jogging back into base allowing the body to cool off. Once back, one should walk around until pulse rate has returned to normal, after which a cool shower followed by a short cold shower should be taken.

Because so much of the game is spent bent off to one side and particularly because players also run in this unbalanced position, low back problems and ham-string injuries are quite a common side effect of this sport. To offset this, extra attention must be paid to the mobility of the low back and a proper stretching, mobilizing and warm-up routine should take place before each game. The programme suggested below is suitable for both men and women and will ensure that, when taking to the field, the areas subjected to the most strain are at their most mobile and, therefore, least liable to injury or strain. It presumes the recommended daily exercises are done as routine.

Exercise and warm up routine
The following exercises are illustrated in the Centre Section.

(Exercise 1)
Hip rotation — repeat 5 times each way.

(Exercise 3)
Trunk twisting — repeat 5 times each way.

(Exercise 2)
Side stretching — repeat 10 times each way.

(Exercise 9)
Alternate leg stretch — repeat 5 times each way.

(Exercise 44)
Sitting leg stretch — repeat 5 times each way.

(Exercise 2)
Side stretching — repeat 10 times each way.

(Exercise 46)
Knee clasp — repeat 10 times each way.

(Exercise 4)
Hands between legs — repeat 10 times.

(Exercise 5)
Jogging on the spot — continue until a general feeling of muscular warmth is achieved (described but not illustrated in Centre Section).

The one-sidedness of the game tends to produce uneven muscular balance in the spine and, to offset this, one-sided exercise should be taken regularly and the simple exercises outlined below should be used to make sure that this compensation is achieved.

Exercises to counteract the one-sidedness of the game (Illustrated in Centre Section)

(Exercise 26)
Side curl — repeat 5 times.

(Exercise 18)
One arm push — repeat 5 times.

(Exercise 25)
Single side stretching — repeat 10 times.

7. RUGBY

Of all the contact sports, rugby is the most totally physical — bringing opposing players into constant aggressive or defensive opposition. The very nature of the game means that a player is liable to meet either an opponent or the ground with considerable force at regular intervals. Injuries in rugby are commonplace, though it has to be said that the average rugby player very rarely leaves the field unless unconscious and carried off!

Whilst certain traumatic injuries are unavoidable, such as cuts, bruises, accidental kicks, etc, at least half the injuries sustained on a rugby field are due to the relative unfitness of the player, and the failure of the player to achieve an adequate standard of health to be able to play the game safely. The character of the typical club rugby player is such that his dietary intake, especially of the liquid form, often leaves a fair amount to be desired! Whilst celebration after a game is very much part of the rugby scene, it is important that, for the largest percentage of the week, a sensible balanced intake of food and drink is maintained. If this is achieved, then the body can cope with the unusual abuse on a Saturday night and, apart from feeling jaded on Sunday morning, there should be little other detrimental effect to the player's ability.

Because rugby contains so much physical contact, it is essential to be in as healthy a state as possible for two reasons. Firstly, the body's ability to absorb impact damage is totally dependent upon the state of the body's chemistry, which determines (a) how serious the injury will become at the moment of impact, and (b) how long it will take to clear up. Unhealthy blood vessels tend to bleed far more when damaged; therefore, bruising is more serious and recovery time is lengthened. Secondly, when less than completely fit, the player's commitment is often less than a hundred per cent, and it is nearly always in these situations that further injury is sustained. To hold back at rugby is to invite further damage.

The medical services available to the typical rugby player are probably the most limited of almost any amateur sport, and many players carry injuries throughout a whole season. The effect of this is to produce long-term damage that, in some cases, may never be totally recovered from. Whilst strength and physical courage are very much part of the game, it is important to make sure that one doesn't lose sight of the old maxim that sometimes 'discretion is the better part of valour'.

The starting point for fitness to play rugby is, of course, pre-season training. The advice given below presumes that the basic instructions outlined earlier in the book are being followed, and builds upon that to produce a sensible physical state at the start of the season. Forwards and backs have to be looked at differently since the nature of their game is very different — though initially, pre-season training for both can be the same. As training progresses, extra work has to be done on stamina for forwards, and speed and agility for the backs. With progress in the modern game it is, however, important, but not always popular, to try to increase the speed and mobility of the pack as a whole. Changes in the rules mean that faster and more agile forwards become a match-winning unit, and to this end they should be encouraged to achieve a higher level of speed and acceleration than has been required previously. Club rugby packs have traditionally carried one or two very large and overweight members whose main job in life is to move from one set scrum to the next set scrum and manage to last out for the eighty minutes!

Besides the sort of traumatic injuries discussed above, which are an inevitable part of the game, and which should be dealt with by having efficient medical advice available on the touch line, there are a vast number of muscular pulls and strains, knee, ankle and arm joint damage, and particularly low back problems, all of which can be laid at the door of inadequate training. Unhealthy muscle tissue leads to a vulnerability to tearing and pulling and, if the spine is not correctly supported by healthy muscle tissue, then it too is liable to sustain damage. The training schedule laid out below is ground-work which should be followed for at least a month before three weeks of different training, dependent on whether or not the player is a forward or a back.

Basic Rugby Training Programme

Players should initially warm themselves up by jogging and moving around. Then the training session proper should commence with the stretching exercises given below. These should be repeated two or three times to make sure that all the players are adequately loosened off, and players should be encouraged to stretch a little further with each exercise.

Warm-up exercises
(Illustrated in Centre Section)

(Exercise 1)
Hip rotation — repeat 5 times each way.
(Exercise 3)
Trunk twisting — repeat 5 times each way.
(Exercise 4)
Hands between legs — commence with 5, build up to 10.
(Exercise 28)
Elbow stretch inhalation — repeat 5 times.
(Exercise 9)
Alternate leg stretch — repeat 5 times each way.
(Exercise 27)
Forced breathing — repeat 5 times.
(Exercise 4)
Hands between legs — repeat 8 times.

The stretching should be followed by jogging on the spot and, from this point on, players should be advised that, unless ordered otherwise, as soon as exercises are finished or a group position is reached, they should continue jogging at all times. This continued movement helps considerably in building stamina, and encourages recovery speed during subsequent matches. The initial burst of jogging should be for about a minute at reasonable speed, after which the stretching exercises should be repeated. After a good stretch, the player should jog on the spot for ten seconds, run on the spot for ten seconds, and repeat this alternation three times.

A third session of stretching exercises should then follow with even greater stretch being achieved by the players. This is followed by three sessions of jogging for ten seconds on the spot, running for ten seconds on the spot and, finally, sprinting for ten seconds on the spot — after which a player should run around the perimeter of a rugby field. During the course of this run, the trainer should suddenly instruct the players to go straight down onto the ground, either on their front or their backs according to command, and to get up immediately on the order 'up'. If people do not respond quickly, it should be repeated until all players react with enthusiasm! By including this in running, it helps the players' ability to regain their feet quickly, which is very valuable during the course of a game.

After two laps with the up and down exercise, group exercise should follow with twenty squat thrusts and twenty leg lifts, with the legs being held together straight and the feet being raised no more than nine inches off the ground. This is followed by twenty head raises with the hands clasped behind the neck and elbows out, and twenty press-ups as summarized below.

Training set exercises
(Illustrated in Centre Section)

(Exercise 58)
Squat thrusts — commence with 10, build up to 20.
(Exercise 51)
Leg lifts — commence with 10, build up to 30.
(Exercise 50)
Chest raises — commence with 10, build up to 30.
(Exercise 55)
Press ups — commence with 10, build up to 30.

Following the set exercises, a 'jog 10, run 10 and sprint 10' session should be undertaken, with subsequent exercises of twenty squat thrusts, twenty press-ups, twenty sit-ups with the legs bent and the hands clasped behind the neck, and twenty star jumps.

Additional set training exercises
(Illustrated in Centre Section)

(Exercise 41)
Sit-ups to both knees — commence with 5, build up to 20.
(Exercise 20)
Squatting star jumps — commence with 6, build up to 15.

These exercises should be followed by two laps of the periphery of the field, with the usual up-and-down interludes, followed by some jogging on the spot and a repeat of the stretching exercises. Shuttle sprints should follow this relaxation period, with ten shuttles of 25 metres, ten shuttles of 40 metres, and ten shuttles of 50 metres, with a short, steady jogging period in between. It is at this point that it is important to make sure that all players continue to commit themselves fully to the exercise, and do not stand still between sprints, as this gives an advantage to the fitter players which, long term, is not to their benefit.

After the shuttles, one lap of the periphery should be completed, followed by a group exercise period again with twenty each of the following exercises in the following pattern: leg raises, head raises, squat thrusts, leg raises (again), press-ups, and twenty star jumps to complete. This should be eased into a gentle jog, keeping people moving the whole time, and as soon as everybody has had a small breathing space, a further twenty (each) squat thrusts, press-ups, and legs-bent sit-ups should follow. A further lap of the periphery of the field, and then a group session of twenty squat thrusts, twenty sit-ups, and ten 'jog, run and sprints' should round off the coached session. The last set of 'jog, run and sprints' should be done to absolute maximum output and can be followed by between three and five laps of the periphery of the field, dependent on the stage of training. At the early part, three laps is sufficient but, after three or four weeks, the distance should be up to five laps. If at the end of five laps players are still looking reasonably fresh, then extra distance can always be added with benefit!

This training programme is listed below in chart form, to make it easier to use by coaches. Coaches should always remember that the average rugby player is not notably keen on training, and in order to help to prevent injury during the season, a touch of the iron fist is generally more effective than the velvet glove.

After the training programme, it is important to cool down properly prior to changing. Cooling down should always be done by walking around while breathing deeply and until pulse returns to a very near normal rate. After this, a shower should be taken — not too hot as this tends to cause sweating to continue — and once one has cooled to blood heat under the shower, a short, sharp cold one, when available, will help peripheral circulation.

After the initial four weeks training, then both forwards and backs should follow a training programme up to the end of Stage 1, and then do the appropriate stage 2 as detailed below.

Rugby Training Programme

Stage 1
Stretching exercises
Jogging on the spot
Stretching exercises
Jog 10 seconds, run 10 seconds (×3)
Stretching exercises
Jog 10 seconds, run 10 seconds, spring 10
   seconds (×3)
2 laps of pitch and up and down discipline
Group exercise:
   20×squat thrusts
   20×9 in leg lifts
   20×head raises
   20×press-ups
Jog 10 seconds, run 10 seconds, sprint 10
   seconds (×3)
Group exercise:
   20×squat thrusts
   20×press-ups
   20×legs-bent sit-ups
   20×star jumps
2 laps of pitch and up and down discipline
Jogging on the spot
Stretching exercises

Stage 2
Shuttle sprints:
   25 metres×10
   40 metres×10
   50 metres×10
1 lap of pitch
Group exercise:
   20×9 in leg raises
   20×head raises
   20×squat thrusts
   20×9 in leg raises
   20×press-ups
   20×star jumps
Jogging on the spot
Group exercise:
   20×squat thrusts
   20×press-ups
   20×legs-bent sit-ups
1 lap of the pitch
Group exercise:
   20×sit-ups
   20×squat thrusts
   Jog 10 seconds, run 10 seconds, sprint 10
     seconds (×3)
3 (or more) laps of the pitch

After the initial pre-season training, a player should move to a more specific training in relation to his particular role in the game and, for this purpose, a suitable training programme is detailed below. All players should do stage 1 of the pre-season training, and then split into forwards and backs for their individual stage 2s.

Backs

The training should commence with a short jogging session to loosen up after the break whilst re-organizing, and be followed by ten 25-metre shuttles, ten 40-metre shuttles, ten 25-metre shuttles and ten 50-metre shuttles with a short period of jogging and breathing in between each set of sprints. These sprints should be followed immediately by a ten second (each) 'jog, run and sprint' session before moving straight into group exercises of twenty press-ups, twenty squat thrusts, twenty leg raises nine inches from the ground, and twenty squat thrusts with a further ten seconds of jogging, running and sprinting, three times.

Following this intense exercise, a period of steady jogging on the spot should be followed by a repeat of the stretching exercises as in stage 1, and then further sprinting from the goal line and the 10-metre line, with a break of ten seconds between each sprint. This should be repeated five times, then players should be divided into teams of between three and five, dependent on numbers available, and a 50-metre relay race, with each player running twice, should then follow. A short breather should be allowed, after which the same teams should then have a two-run relay for the full length of the pitch. The more equally balanced the teams can be made, then of course the more effective the competition that takes place.

After the relay, a good team game to help handling and speed is to space the players equally down the pitch, standing with their backs to the starting point, with the first player taking the ball in his hands on the goal line. At the whistle, the player runs to the player ahead of him who should bend forward, the runner then rolls the ball between his team-mate's legs, who picks it up, sprints to the next player in front of him, rolls the ball through and so on, until the last player touches down at the far goal line, turns round, runs the length of the pitch and recommences the process until every player has completed the revolution twice. Once the ball-game is completed, there should be a 50-metre relay, again with the same teams, and then everybody participates in ten 25-metre shuttles at maximum pace. To round off, jog for ten seconds, run for ten seconds and sprint for ten seconds, three times, all at absolute maximum effort, before a final three or more laps of the pitch to end the training.

The backs' stage 2 training programme is tabulated below for ease of use:

Backs — *Stage 2*
Jog
Shuttles:
   25 metres×10
   Jog
   40 metres×10
   Jog
   25 metres×10
   Jog
   50 metres×10
1 lap of the pitch
Jog 10 seconds, run 10 seconds, sprint 10 seconds (×3)
Group exercise:
   20×press-ups
   20×squat thrusts

20×9 in leg raises
20×squat thrusts
Jog 10 seconds, run 10 seconds, sprint 10
  seconds (×3)
Jogging on the spot
Stretching exercises
Sprints to 10-metre line with 10 second
  break (×5)
50-metre relay
Full length pitch relay
Ball rolling game
50-metre relay
Shuttles:
  25 metres×10
Jog 10 seconds, run 10 seconds, sprint 10
  seconds (maximum effort)
3 laps (or more) of the pitch

Forwards

Stage 2 training for the forwards should commence with a gentle jog, after the re-organization of the players. Then players should be split into pairs and the back-to-back double lift (Exercise 47, Centre Section) should be done five times and held for a period of twenty seconds on each particular lift. It is important to match players of nearly equal height and weight, so that both players achieve the same benefit, and collapse is unlikely.

The lift is followed by a series of group exercises, consisting of twenty squat thrusts, twenty leg lifts to nine inches, twenty sit-ups with the legs bent, twenty press-ups, twenty head raises, a further twenty squat thrusts and twenty sit-ups, and twenty nine-inch leg raises. This pattern is followed by jogging for ten seconds and running for ten seconds on the spot, repeated three times.

Two laps of the field with the up and down discipline should then be undertaken, with jogging on the spot followed by a period of stretching, using the exercises as in stage 1.

The players should then be divided into teams of between three and five people, dependent on the number available, and a leap-frog relay should follow. Players are spaced equally down the field, back to the starting point, in the bent position with hands on the knees, the first runner starts at the goal line and vaults over his team mates on the way to the far goal line, then returns to the starting point before releasing the next runner. Each player should repeat this revolution twice. Then the same teams should compete in a relay the full length of the pitch and back, again each player completing it twice. Individual players should then do ten 25-metre shuttles, followed by ten 50-metre shuttles. Jogging on the spot follows, before the commencement of a group exercise of twenty squat thrusts, twenty star jumps, twenty knees-bent sit-ups, and twenty press-ups. One lap of the pitch with the up and down discipline should be taken at a fair pace, then the last group exercise of twenty star jumps, twenty squat thrusts, twenty press-ups, twenty nine-inch leg raises, and a 'jog, run and sprint' session at maximum pace is followed by three or more laps of the field to end the training programme.

The programme is tabulated below for ease of use, and very few forwards who successfully complete this programme will disgrace themselves fitness-wise during the ensuing season.

Forwards — *Stage 2*
Jogging on the spot
Group exercise:
  Double lift, 20 seconds (×5)
  20×squat thrusts
  20×9 in leg lifts
  20×legs-bent sit-ups
  20×press-ups

20×head raises
20×squat thrusts
20×sit-ups
20×9 in leg raises
Jog 10 seconds, run 10 seconds (×3)
2 laps of the pitch and up and down discipline
Jogging on the spot
Stretching
Leap-frog game
Full pitch relay
Shuttles:
    25 metres×10
    50 metres×10
Jogging on the spot
Group exercise:
    20×squat thrusts
    20×star jumps
    20×legs-bent sit-ups
    20×press-ups
1 lap of the pitch and up and down discipline
Group exercise:
    20×star jumps
    20×squat thrusts
    20×press-ups
    20×9 in leg raises
Jog 10 seconds, run 10 seconds, sprint 10 seconds (at maximum effort) (×3)

In addition to the general training outlined above and club training, each player should run at least twice a week for a minimum of thirty minutes at a steady pace in relation to his own particular speed. The pace of the running should be steadily increased from the start so that maximum speed is reached about fifteen minutes into the run and maintained for about ten minutes, before a gradual five minutes slow down to the end of the run to allow the body to get back to a steady rhythm of breathing and pulse.

After any training session or any run, cooling down is important and should certainly not be overlooked, as failure to cool down properly can lead to stiffness and tightness in muscle tissues which can result in eventual damage. As soon as the training or the running is finished, walk around steadily, breathe in deeply until such time as pulse and heart feel normal, the breathing is steady, and sweating has steadied down. One should also put something warm around the upper body to prevent any unduly rapid chilling taking place. Once this state has been achieved, then a warm rather than hot shower should be taken and, whenever possible, a cold spray to finish helps to stimulate the circulation, tone up the skin state, and help to prevent any further problems with aches and stiffness in the muscles.

Most club teams have their own warm-up routine before a game which usually consists of fairly energetic arm and leg swinging exercises, and jogging and running on the spot. Whilst this is fine as a pre-match circulatory stimulator, every player should spend at least five–six minutes stretching off, prior to doing this team warm up. The simple stretching exercises outlined below should always be done before any game, and will help to ensure that most of the muscular damage which can occur during a game will be avoided. These stretching exercises should never be forced but should be relaxed into, allowing the muscles to steadily stretch as the body's own weight takes its effect.

Stretching exercises
(Illustrated in Centre Section)

(Exercise 9)
Alternate leg stretch — repeat 5 times each way.
(Exercise 44)
Sitting leg stretch — repeat 5 times each way.
(Exercise 46)
Knee clasp — repeat 5 times each way.

(Exercise 4)
Hands between legs — repeat 5 times.

Once the season has started, it is still important to maintain fitness, and stage 1 of the general training programme should be completed at least once a week by all players and, as the season progresses, ball handling exercises will keep adding to the general level of sharpness and ability of each player.

It must be emphasized that the physical input into these training sessions must be of the highest level, or otherwise one is only fooling oneself as to the level of fitness attained. If a player does not feel thoroughly exhausted at the end of a session then it is fair to say that he has not committed himself to the best of his ability. The only person who suffers by such a lack of commitment is the player himself.

To those who sustain injuries during a game, the best advice is always, 'if in doubt don't play on'. Whilst team spirit may appear to dictate that one should continue to play at all cost, particularly where no substitutes are available, common sense and body awareness advise the opposite. Many problems which would involve perhaps one week recovery periods, become four and five week injuries because of further damage due to continued play.

All rugby clubs should try to contact a physiotherapist, an osteopath and a sports-injury interested doctor in their area and to open lines of communication with them, in order to establish an injury treatment service for their players. If these services can be made available, then many players who might otherwise spend many games on the bench, will end up having a full and satisfying season.

8. SOCCER

The modern game of soccer, despite recent controversies, is still considered by many to be the British national sport. As with almost all sports, the speed of the game has increased dramatically and correspondingly higher fitness levels are demanded.

Both amateur and professional football training has, for many years in many clubs, followed a very similar basic pattern. Despite the huge amounts of money invested in soccer, a large proportion of teams still have very antiquated training routines. One of the main ideas of soccer training appears to be to produce players with tremendous quads (the muscles at the front of the thigh) which are the hallmark of a footballer, with the necessary tight fitting trousers! The production of these muscles seems to be at the expense of body balance as a whole, and even first division clubs are prone to this sort of oversight in training routine.

A few years ago, a leading club had a training routine which involved a tremendous amount of development of the quads, at the expense of mobility of the hip and knee joint, all the strengthening exercises being done over short-range movements. The net result of this training was that, because of the compensatory tightening in the ham-strings (the muscles at the back of the thigh) the club suffered seventeen ham-string injuries to various players during the course of the season. This problem was not the bad luck that the club thought it to be, but purely the result of archaic and unconsidered training. Muscle strength should never be increased at the expense of mobility, particularly in an area

which is the main functional zone in the sport concerned.

A lot of amateur soccer players, and a surprising number of professionals, are nowhere near as fit on an all-body basis as they should be. Apart from low back and leg problems due to unbalanced development of the lower body in relation to the upper body, inadequate out-of-club training is usually to blame for the problems that arise. There are, of course, traumatic injuries that result from trips, falls and direct impact, and these are dealt with in the final chapter.

Every player should undertake a running programme off their own bat outside their normal training, and a minimum target should be twenty minutes twice per week, consisting of five minutes steady running, ten minutes faster pace running with occasional sprints, and five minutes steady running prior to returning to base. After the run, stretching exercises as in the daily routine should be used to make sure no long-term tightness occurs, and the player should walk around until pulse returns to normal, after which a body-heat shower or bath followed by a cold shower or splash should be taken. This running and subsequent sport presumes that the basic dietary and exercise advice outlined in the earlier chapters is followed as, without reasonable body state at commencement, no training programme can be either safe or effective.

Pre-season training is obviously important since, without this, not only can one not play the game effectively but one is vulnerable to stretch and strain injuries and more liable to receive traumatic injury as the body will not be sufficiently elastic and stable to effectively resist external pressures. A suitable pre-season training routine which should be undertaken at least twice per week should start off with the stretching exercises outlined here and illustrated in the Centre Section.

Stretching exercises
(Illustrated in Centre Section)

(Exercise 1)
Hip rotation — repeat 10 times each way.
(Exercise 3)
Trunk twisting — repeat 10 times each way.
(Exercise 2)
Side stretching — repeat 10 times each way.
(Exercise 4)
Hands between legs — repeat 10 times.
(Exercise 46)
Knee clasp — commence with 10, build up to 20.
(Exercise 28)
Elbow stretch inhalation — repeat 10 times.
(Exercise 9)
Alternate leg stretch — repeat until tired.
(Exercise 46)
Knee clasp — repeat 10 times each way.
(Exercise 4)
Hands between legs — repeat 10 times.
(Exercise 9)
Alternate leg stretch — repeat three or four times more.

These exercises should be followed by jogging on the spot at a steady pace, but lifting the knees well, for about 60-90 seconds, with a one-minute session of running on the spot to follow. The stretching exercises should then be repeated, each one being done at least five times, with more and more steady pressure into each stretch without forcing it.

The initial warm-up should then be followed by two laps of the periphery of the football pitch, at a steady but certainly not a slow pace. A break should then be taken to jog for ten seconds on the spot, run for ten seconds on the spot, and then sprint for ten seconds on the spot, which exercise should be repeated three times prior to a further two laps at a slightly higher pace round the periphery of the pitch. The player should then find adequate space to move arms and legs freely, and the following group exercises should be done: twenty squat thrusts, twenty nine-inch leg raises, twenty salmon raises, twenty nine-inch leg raises (with the legs being opened and closed twice before lowering), twenty press-ups, twenty legs-bent sit-ups, twenty squat thrusts, and twenty nine-inch leg raises. Jogging, running and sprinting for ten seconds each on the spot should then be repeated three times.

A further two laps of the pitch should be completed again at a slightly higher pace with five series of stretching exercises to follow. Group exercise should then take place with players splitting into pairs to do twenty fixed ankle lifts on first the right leg and then the left leg, then twenty fixed ankle lifts on both legs. All players should then exercise individually, with twenty knees to chest and squeeze, twenty knees-bent sit-ups, twenty salmon raises, twenty nine-inch leg raises opening and closing twice, and twenty squat thrusts. A further lap of the pitch should be followed by group exercise of twenty squatting star jumps, twenty hops on the right leg, twenty on the left leg, twenty bounces as high as possible on both legs, twenty squat thrusts and twenty further fixed ankle lifts with both legs.

A further couple of minutes of steady jogging and breathing, followed by stretching exercises, should then lead into ten

25-metre shuttle sprints, a short breather, and then ten 50-metre shuttle sprints, followed by group exercises of twenty nine-inch leg raises, and the same number each of press-ups, legs-bent sit-ups and squat thrusts. A final session of jogging, running and sprinting on the spot for ten seconds each is repeated three times with a maximum effort on the last sprint. The training should round off with three laps round the periphery of the pitch and deep breathing and walking around after the last lap until pulse has returned to normal. These exercises are illustrated in the Centre Section. A body-heat shower and, where possible, a cold spray to finish should then be taken to complete the session.

Set training routine
(Exercises are illustrated in the Centre Section)

(Exercise 58)
Squat thrusts — commence with 10, build up to 30.
(Exercise 51)
Leg lifts — commence with 10, build up to 30.
(Exercise 52)
Salmon raise — commence with 10, build up to 30.
(Exercise 57)
Leg raise 9 in, open and close — commence with 5, build up to 15.
(Exercise 55)
Press-ups — commence with 10, build up to 30.
(Exercise 41)
Sit-ups to both knees — commence with 10, build up to 30.
(Exercise 59)
Ankle-restrained leg lift — repeat with each leg.

(Exercise 60)
Double-ankle restrained leg lift — continue effort for a count of 3.
(Exercise 46)
Knee clasp — repeat 10 times.
(Exercise 20)
Squatting star jumps — commence with 10, build up to 30.
(Exercise 7)
Hopping — repeat 10 times (described but not illustrated in Centre Section).
(Exercise 8)
Bouncing — repeat 10 times (described but not illustrated in Centre Section).

Competitive relays and sprints may also be included in the programme, once training has reached a reasonable point and then, of course, ball skills and ball training programmes will increase the variety and the type of work undertaken at the coach's discretion.

Soccer Programme Summary

Stretching exercises
Jogging on the spot
Running on the spot
Stretching exercises
2 laps of the pitch
Jog 10 seconds, run 10 seconds, sprint 10 seconds (×3)
2 laps of the pitch
Group exercise:
   20×squat thrusts
   20×9 in leg raises
   20×salmon raises
   20×9 in leg raises (open and close twice)
   20×press-ups
   20×legs-bent sit-ups
   20×squat thrusts
   20×9 in leg raises
Jog 10 seconds, run 10 seconds, sprint 10 seconds (×3)

2 laps of the pitch
Stretching exercises
Group exercise:
    20×fixed ankle leg lifts (alternate legs)
    20×fixed ankle leg lifts (both legs)
    20×knees to chin and squeeze
    20×salmon raises
    20×9 in leg lifts (open and close twice)
    20×squat thrusts
1 lap of the pitch
Group exercise:
    20×squatting star jumps
    20×hops (right leg)
    20×hops (left leg)
    20×bounces (both legs)
    20×squat thrusts
    20×fixed ankle leg lifts (both legs)
Jogging on the spot
Stretching exercises
Shuttles:
    10×25 metre
    10×50 metre
Group exercise:
    20×9 in leg raises
    20×press-ups
    20×legs-bent sit-ups
    20×squat thrusts
Jog 10 seconds, run 10 seconds, sprint 10
    seconds (×3)
3 laps of the pitch
Cool down

Whilst the above programme will prepare the player for the season, it is important to realize that, although playing takes a more important part once the season is underway, consistent running and training must be continued during the season if the level of fitness is not to fall off. Very little of the above programme should be reduced during the season: instead skilled work and other training should be included on top because, the greater the level of fitness, the better the standard of play and the less the chance of injury during the course of playing. When injuries are sustained during the course of football, particularly knee injuries which are very prevalent in the sport, it is important to get suitable advice as soon as is possible. The use of anti-inflammatory injections and pain-killing drugs and sprays in order to allow a player to continue for an important game has resulted in many retired footballers having painful or chronically arthritic knee problems. For the amateur, especially, it is always advisable to seek advice if in any doubt as to whether or not one is fit to play.

Every club of an amateur status should ensure that it has access to a physiotherapist, a doctor with an interest in sports medicine and certainly wherever possible, an osteopath similarly inclined. If the combined skills of these three practitioners are available, then players should be able to obtain rapid and accurate diagnosis, rapid and effective advice on whether to play or when to play and, above all, the right treatment rapidly applied.

9. BASKETBALL AND NETBALL

Netball has long been a popular game in Britain, and in recent years basketball has developed a hugely increased following. Although there are, of course, differences between the two sports, the basic fitness requirements are very similar and, therefore, can be dealt with jointly from the point of view of a basic training programme to achieve a level where the individual skills can be developed.

A high level of stamina, explosive power and mobility are required in order to be able to play either of the two sports, and to this end the basic fitness advice and regular running are an important part of developing the starting point for specific training. A run of twenty–thirty minutes duration should be taken at least three times a week, with the first and last five minutes of the run being at a steadier pace, and with the run preceded and followed by the back mobility exercises outlined here.

Back mobility exercises
(Illustrated in Centre Section)

(Exercise 37)
Cat stretch — commence with 10, build up to 30.
(Exercise 38)
Forehead to knee — commence with 10, build up to 30.
(Exercise 39)
Opposite arm and leg stretch — commence with 10, build up to 20.
(Exercise 1)
Hip rotation — repeat 10 times each way.

(Exercise 3)
Trunk twisting — repeat 10 times each way.
(Exercise 49)
Abdominal press — commence with 20, build up to 30.
(Exercise 53)
Alternate knee raises — repeat 10 times with each knee.
(Exercise 37)
Cat stretch — commence with 10, build up to 20.
(Exercise 4)
Hands between legs — repeat 10 times.

After the exercises, a cool shower should then be taken with, where possible, a short, sharp, cold shower to finish off.

A pre-season training programme should be undertaken, and this should be based on steady running with short, sharp shuttle sprints included, and should be done on the days when a regular run is not used. After the run and the sprints, the following specific exercise programme should be done to develop the required muscular structures and maintain the mobility that is required to successfully compete in either sport.

Basketball and Netball Training Programme

Jog 10 seconds on spot
Run 10 seconds on spot
Jog 10 seconds on spot
Run 10 seconds on spot
Hip circle

Hip rotation
Side bend
Hands between legs
Leg stretch
Knees to chest
Jog 10 seconds on spot
Run 10 seconds on spot
Sprint 10 seconds on spot
Side bend
10 press-ups
10 knees-bent sit-ups
10 salmon raises
10 knees to chest and hug
10 squat thrusts
Jog 10 seconds on spot
Run 10 seconds on spot
Sprint 10 seconds on spot
20 hops (right leg)
20 hops (left leg)
20 bounces (on both legs)
10 squatting star jumps
20 squat thrusts
10 press-ups
20 9 in leg raises
20 salmon raises
10 knees to chest and hug
Jog 10 seconds on spot
Run 10 seconds on spot
Sprint 10 seconds on spot
20 squatting star jumps
20 hops (right leg)
20 hops (left leg)
20 bounces (both legs)
20 knees-up jumps
20 press-ups
20 salmon raises
20 squat thrusts
Jog 10 seconds on spot
Run 10 seconds on spot
Sprint 10 seconds on spot
Then 5 minutes steady running to cool down.

During the season and so long as the regular running is followed, the above exercise programme should be done on the days when a run is not undertaken. The combination of this with the specific coaching which is part of the game should ensure that any injuries sustained will not be of a self-inflicted nature due to lack of fitness.

In basketball in particular, ankles can be vulnerable because of pushing and barging and the difficulty of always landing square on the feet. If any damage has been sustained, it is sensible always to tape the ankle and properly reinforce it so that further damage does not ensue. In many clubs in America, players are forced by contract to tape ankles in order to avoid their inability to play due to injuries from that source. An effective ankle strapping can be found in the treatments chapter and, if in any doubt, should always be used. If ankle injury has been sustained, then the simple exercises given will help to strengthen the joint in the shortest possible time.

Exercises for ankle injuries
(Description in Centre Section)

(Exercise 30)
Ankle raise — continue until tired.
(Exercise 31)
Ankle flex and extend — continue until tired.

Owing to the highly competitive nature of the two sports, a number of traumatic injuries can be sustained and, if play is continued whilst carrying these injuries, the effects can become both painful and long-term. It is sensible for all teams or clubs to arrange contacts with physiotherapists, osteopaths and chiropractors in their area, as this type of treatment is very necessary, particularly the more professional the approach becomes.

Players should always remember to make sure a good warm-up takes place before each game, and that mobility exercises are done after a game to make sure that no stiffness is carried forward to subsequent training and the next game. A simple routine for pre- and post-match is outlined below.

Pre- and post-match exercises
(Illustrated in Centre Section)

(Exercise 37)
Cat stretch — repeat 15 times, building up to 25 times.
(Exercise 49)
Abdominal press — repeat 25 times.
(Exercise 46)
Knee clasp — commence with 5, build up to 20.

(Exercise 44)
Sitting leg stretch — repeat 10 times each side.
(Exercise 42)
Hip stretch — repeat 5 times each side.
(Exercise 37)
Cat stretch — repeat 10 times.
(Exercise 4)
Hands between legs — repeat 10 times.

The ability to obtain pleasure from basketball and netball is dependent on being able to compete consistently in what are surprisingly physical sports. This can only happen if adequate time and effort is made in pre-coaching training to allow the body to absorb the stresses and strains which occur during the course of a match.

EXERCISE SECTION

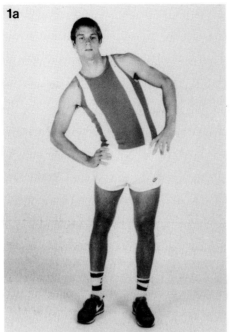

1a

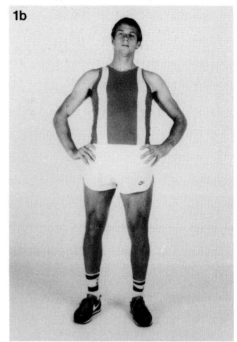

1b

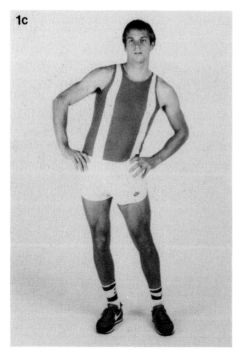

1c

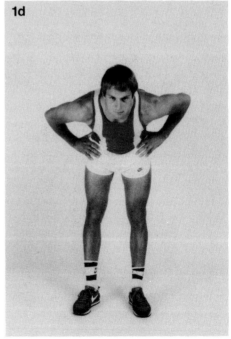

1d

Exercise 1. Hip Rotation

With feet apart, hands on the hips and knees unlocked, the whole pelvic girdle is pushed in a complete circle in both directions. It is important not to lock the knees as this prevents the range of movement which is necessary to fully mobilize and exercise the low back.

Exercise 2. Side Stretching

With feet comfortably apart, knees unlocked and back straight, the left arm is slid down the left leg whilst the right arm curls over the top of the head. It is important not to lean forward during this exercise, as it completely alters the overall effect.

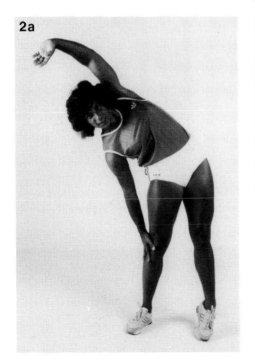

2a

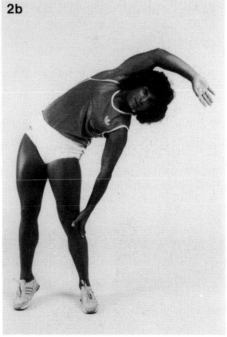

2b

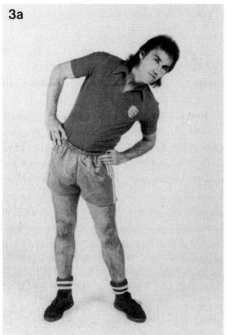

3a

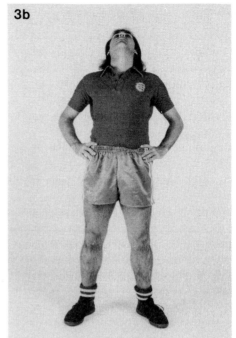

3b

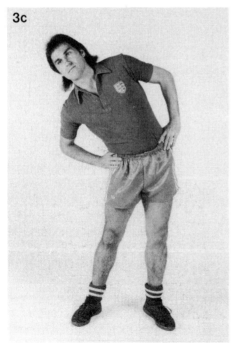

3c

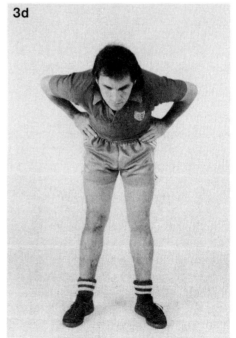

3d

Exercise 3. Trunk Twisting

With the feet comfortably apart, the hands on the hips and knees not locked, the body above the waistline is circled in a complete movement in both directions. It is important not to lock the knees as this increases strain on the low back.

Exercise 4. Hands Between Legs

Begin with feet well apart, knees slightly bent and in the upright position, then bend from the waist and let the hands relax on a line with the feet, and stretch towards the ground. Bob gently to increase the stretching and then straighten back to the commencing position. After repeating this three times, the hands should then be taken further back through the legs with the same process of stretching repeated. Never do this exercise with the knees locked and do not force the amount of rearward stretch. As body mobility increases, the range of stretch will become greater, but some people will never be anatomically capable of reaching the ground comfortably or having a major stretch in the rearward position.

4a

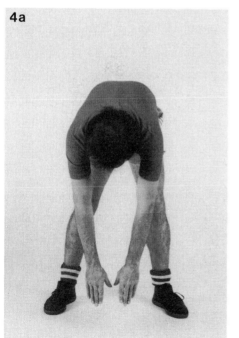

4b

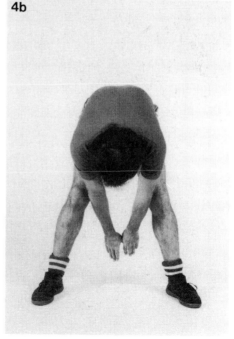

Exercise 5. Jogging and Running on the Spot

Jogging means a reasonable pace of leg movement on the spot, and it should be done with a good, high, knee-lifting action. With the running on the spot, the pace should be increased considerably, but not to the level of an actual sprint. Make sure that whilst jogging or running that one stays as stationary as possible and use the arms as well as just the legs.

Exercise 6. Jog and Hop

The jogging should be on the spot with a good knee lift and a steady arm action, and should last long enough to cause a reasonable degree of cardiovascular stimulation, ie, breathlessness and an increase in pulse rate. This should then be followed by hopping on the spot on each leg in turn. Make the hop as powerful as possible, with a particular effort to drive upwards in the air with the ankle straightening out on take-off. This will greatly increase the ability of the player to jump when required on the court.

Exercise 7. Hopping

Hop on each leg in turn, making sure that as much height as possible is gained in the hop with good ankle extension, and try to land as carefully as possible in a controlled fashion. It greatly improves ankle strength and body balance if every effort is made to keep this exercise carefully controlled.

Exercise 8. Bouncing

This is equivalent to hopping on both feet together and, once again, maximum height and maximum control should be the object of the exercise.

Exercise 9. Alternate Leg Stretch

Commencing in the illustrated position, gradually apply extra pressure to the forward movement, until maximum comfortable stretch is achieved. Then, without moving the feet, turn round and repeat the exercise in the opposite direction. As greater mobility is achieved, then an actual lunge into the stretch position can gradually be employed.

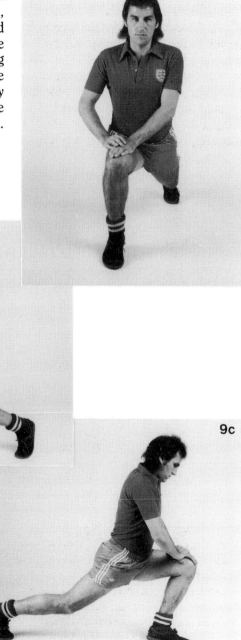

9a

9b

9c

Exercise 10. Arm Stretch

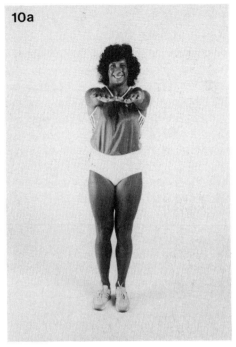

10a

The commencing position is taken up as illustrated and the whole shoulder girdle is moved through a complete arc in either direction. It is important to make this movement as full as possible as this improves mobility around the neck and shoulder area.

Exercise 11. Neck Stretch

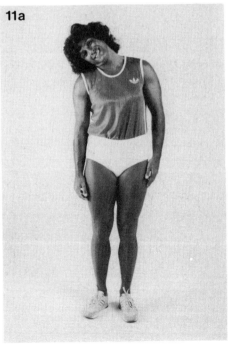

11a

Stretch the head over to the right side and try to increase the movement by letting the restraining muscles relax, allowing the head to fall over as far as possible. Then repeat this to the left side. Next, stretch the chin towards the chest, again allow relaxation of the controlling muscles and achieve as much forward movement as possible, and then slowly take the head back over the centre point and let it drop back, using the weight of the head as the stretching mechanism. Finally, holding the chin to the right, let the head roll in a semi-circle across the front of the body and finish up on the left — repeat this with the same semi-circle to the back. Do not take the head in a full circle as it is possible, whilst doing this, to cause some discomfort in the neck itself.

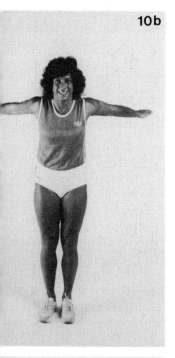

10b

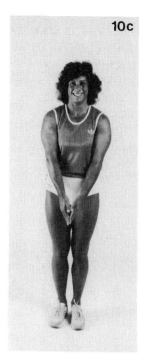

10c

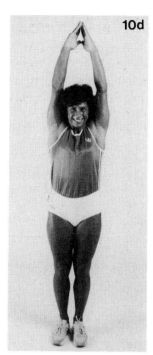

10d

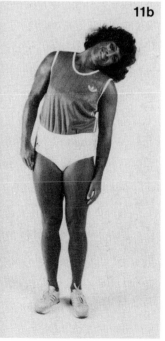

11b

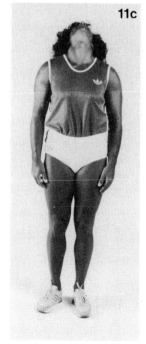

11c

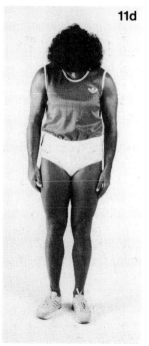

11d

Exercise 12. Shoulder Shrugs

The important thing whilst doing this exercise is to make sure that shoulders are raised as fully as possible and then rotated to the maximum potential range through the whole circle. Whilst there may be some initial discomfort whilst undertaking this movement, this will soon disappear as mobility increases. This particular movement is very effective in helping to avoid potential shoulder damage due to restriction whilst stretching for shots or serving in the game of tennis.

Exercise 13. Arm Flex with Weight

Using any convenient and relatively light weight, eg, a bag of sugar as in the illustration, move the arm slowly through the arc illustrated and concentrate on making the muscles work whilst doing the exercise. To watch in a mirror and to direct the attention to the muscles under use often helps to increase the effectiveness of the exercise. As the power increases, then the size of the weight should steadily be increased and the pace of the exercise slowed down. Whilst dumb-bells can be used as weights when available, there are many objects of convenient size and shape that can be equally effective — ie, bags of sugar or flour, potato snacks, etc.

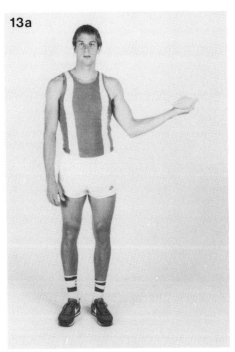

13a

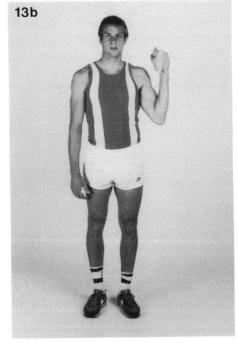

13b

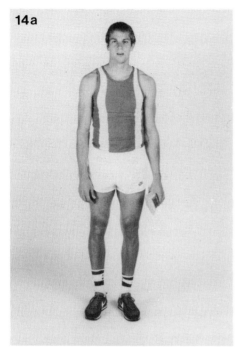 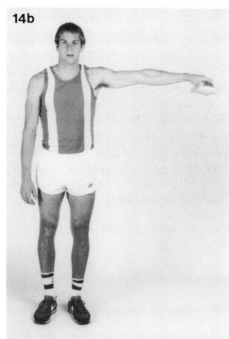

Exercise 14.
Arm Exercise Using Weight

As in the previous exercise, commence with the lighter weights and at a steady speed, and increase the amount of weight and decrease the pace as the muscle becomes more powerful.

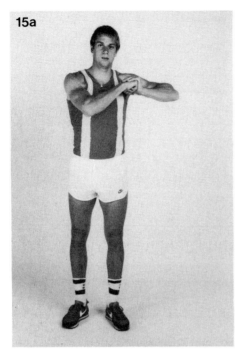

15a

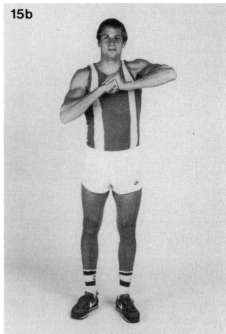

15b

Exercise 15.
Contra-pressure Exercise

This exercise is best done where a mirror is available as this facilitates concentration of the effort on the muscles being used. As can be seen, one hand is pushed into the palm of the other and the opposite hand's resistance is used to get maximum possible effort out of the arm being exercised. The movement from position one to position two should be very slow and steady and the exercise may be repeated until some degree of muscle fatigue is felt.

Exercise 16.
Contra-pressure Exercise

As with exercise 15, this is once again best undertaken in front of a mirror, the importance of slow, steady movement cannot be over-estimated. Concentrate the effort in the arm being exercised, and increase the number of exercises as body strength increases.

16a

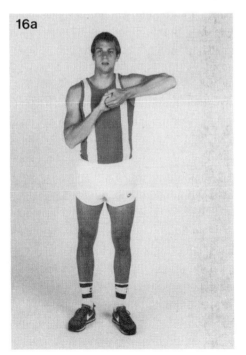

16b

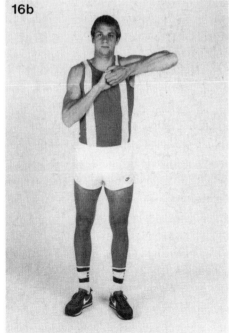

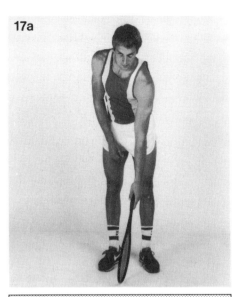

17a

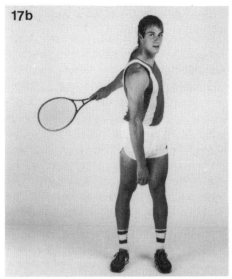

17b

Exercise 17. Racquet Swing

This exercise should be followed to the full range of swing available, and obviously needs adequate space to avoid damage. It is important to let the swing build up as movement is continued, and to try to create a rhythm which makes the exercise far more effective. It should be continued until there is a feeling of warmth in the muscle and a physical awareness of some exercise having taken place. The more tennis or racquet sport that has been played in the preceding period of time, the longer the session of this particular exercise should be.

Exercise 18. One Arm Push

In the early stages of exercising, this exercise should be done as shown here with the feet reasonably close to the wall. The pressure should be steady and not rushed, and should be from full bend to full stretch. As the arm becomes stronger, the feet can be moved further and further from the wall which increases the amount of effort required to undertake the movement.

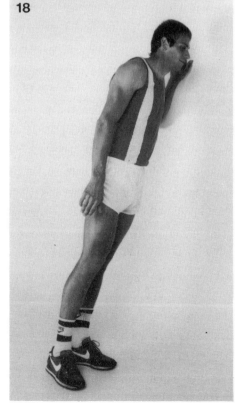

18

Exercise 19. Wall Push and Rotate

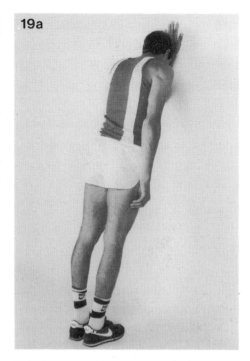

19a

Commence in the position shown, leaning against the wall with feet firmly planted, and with all the weight resting on the arm. Then straighten the arm out, at the same time rotating the body around, but keep the feet firmly anchored on the floor. As the arm strength increases, the feet may be moved further from the wall to increase the amount of pressure placed on the exercise. This exercise is, of course, only done with the arm not normally used in the course of the game.

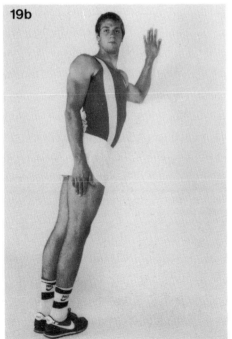

19b

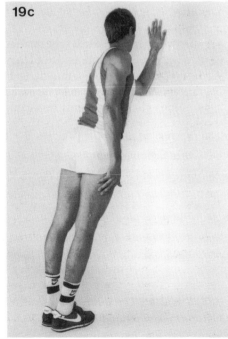

19c

20a

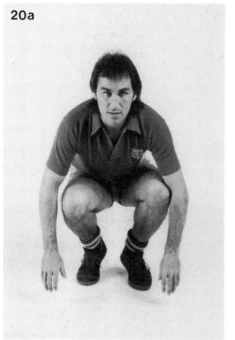

20b

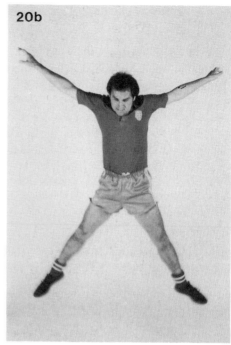

Exercise 20. Squatting Star Jumps

Starting in the position shown in the illustration, a full-blooded jump is required to get sufficient height to achieve the second position illustrated, prior to landing back down and straight back to the starting position.

Exercise 21. Shrugging

The object of this is to pull the shoulders up as close to the ears as possible and then rotate in a full circle. Once the circuit is completed in one direction, the movement should be completed in the opposite direction.

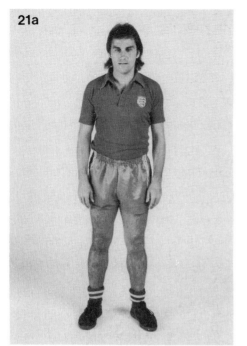

21a

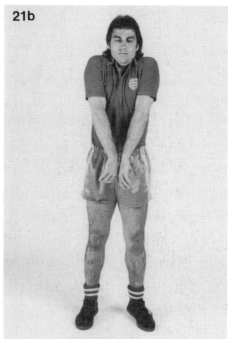

21b

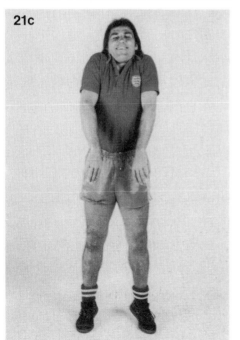

21c

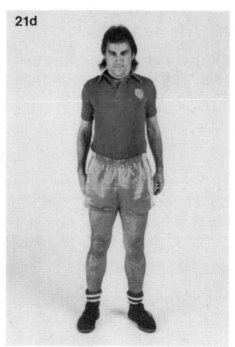

21d

Exercise 22. Arm Swing

This exercise for racquet sports involves swinging the non-playing arm in a complete circle in both directions and repeating about half a dozen times until the arm swings freely and without restriction.

Exercise 23. Alternate Arm Swinging

Standing upright with knees slightly bent, commence by swinging the arm in a forward and upwards direction: scrape the ear on the way past, and swing around the back as far as possible. Then repeat this with the opposite arm. The cycle should then be repeated. It is important to make sure that the swing is as full as possible and that the rest of the body is not moving around whilst the arms are being exercised.

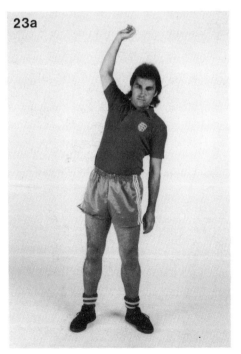

23a

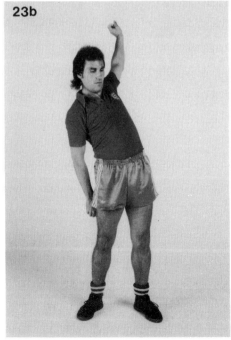

23b

Exercise 24. Double Arm Swing

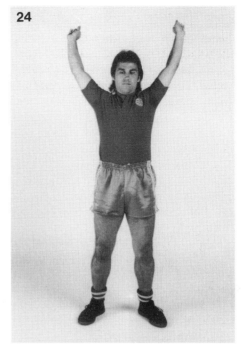

24

Both arms should be swung in a simultaneous direction for a full circle, and then the process repeated in the opposite direction.

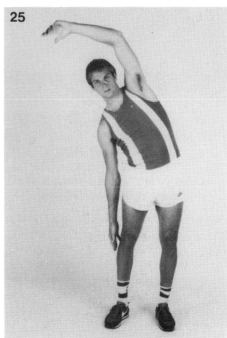

25

Exercise 25. Single Side Stretching

Commence the exercise as illustrated, reaching with the arm as far as possible, making sure that the knees are slightly bent and that, above all, the back is straight and not leaning forwards.

Exercise 26. Side Curl

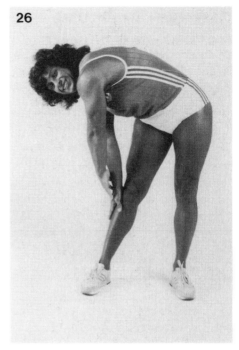

26

The exercise is done as shown, the bending and stretching being purely and simply done to the left side to compensate for the normal angle of the game of hockey.

Exercise 27. Forced Breathing

With feet apart, knees slightly bent, take in a steady deep breath, straighten to the upright position as shown in the illustration. Hold the breath for a count of two and then exhale, relaxing and flopping down to the original starting position.

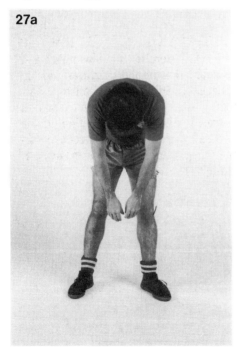

27a

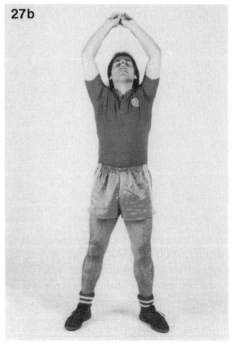

27b

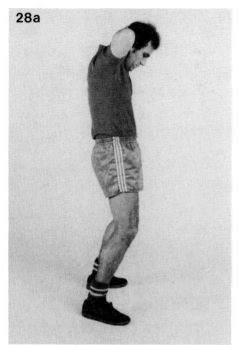

28a

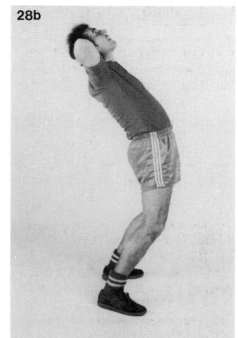

28b

Exercise 28.
Elbow Stretch Inhalation

Commence exercise as in illustration and inhale, allowing the abdomen to extend and the base of the rib-cage to stretch on the in-breath, with the elbows coming up as illustrated in the second illustration. On the out-breath, deflate the abdomen, let the rib-cage collapse and relax back to the original starting position.

Exercise 29. Wall Stretch

Get in as close to the wall as possible as illustrated. Straighten the legs up the wall and keep them there for a count of 20. As mobility in the hips improves, one should be able to get closer and closer to the wall with the legs completely straight and knees locked up against the wall.

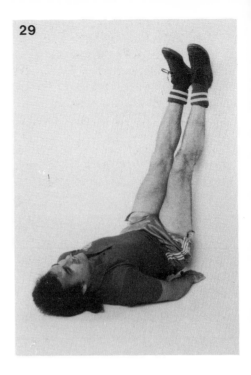

Exercise 30. Ankle Raise

With all the weight on the bad ankle, raise gently up to full stretch and then lower down, keeping the back as straight as possible whilst the exercise is undertaken. This should be continued until the ankle muscle is too tired to continue.

Exercise 31. Ankle Flex and Extend

Standing on the edge of the stair, slowly lower down over the edge taking the bulk of the weight on the bad ankle, and lowering as far as is possible. From this point, raise up onto the toes until maximum stretch is obtained, once again using the bad ankle for the bulk of the effort. As ankle strength increases, this may eventually be done on the one ankle only.

Exercise 32. Knee Exercising

The main object of this exercise is to get as much movement in every direction from the knees, whilst, at the same time, making the muscles work as much as possible.

Try to gradually increase the range of movement and make it more controlled and slower as knee strength increases. It should be steadily possible to make the exercise more and more effective by increased range of movement.

32a

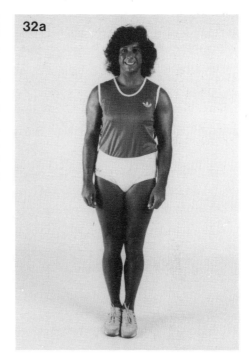

32b

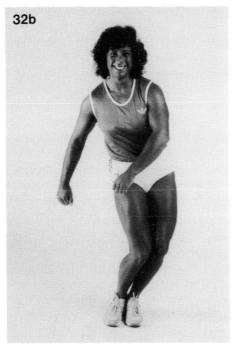

32c

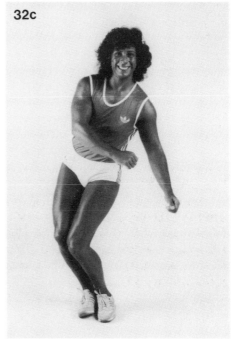

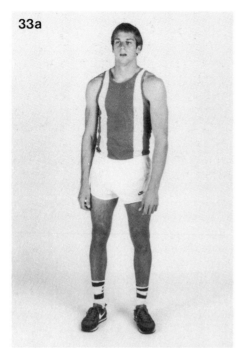

33a

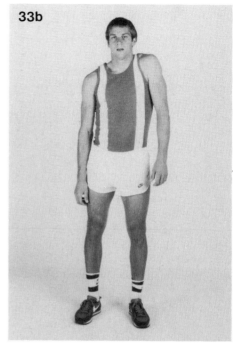

33b

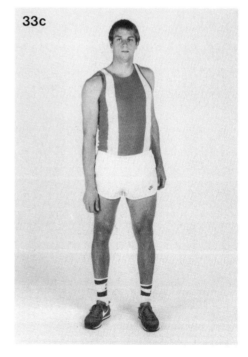

33c

Exercise 33. Shoulder Swing

It is important when rotating the arms as shown here to make sure that the rotation is to the full extent available, and that the initial movement is not forced. As the shoulders gradually become looser and more mobile, then greater pressure can be put upon the swing to increase the range of movement even further.

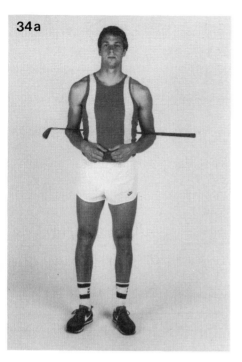

34a

Exercise 34.
Back Turn Using Golf Club

The arms should be comfortably hooked around the golf club, feet placed apart, the knees slightly bent, and the rotation should be as much as is possible until early signs of stress are felt. As mobility increases, greater force can be applied steadily to the rotation and this, in turn, will improve upon the original mobility.

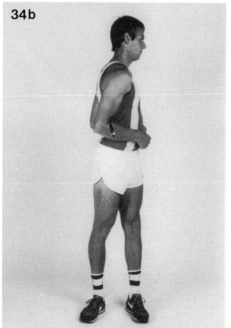

34b

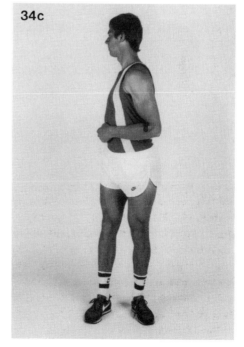

34c

35a

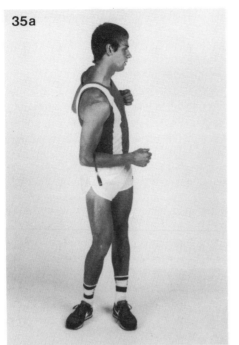

35b

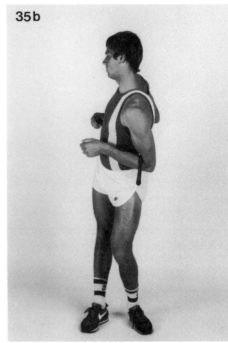

Exercise 35.
Swing and Turn Using Golf Club

Commence with the feet apart and knees slightly bent and rotate and dip as shown, with steady pressure initially, building up a little as the movement becomes easier. After a period of time, when body mobility is increased, the amount of pressure and movement can steadily increase. This exercise is particularly beneficial as it helps nearly all the muscles involved in the turn, rotation and hip movement necessary to strike a golf ball correctly.

Exercise 36. Hip Swing

Commence in the position illustrated and then stretch to the second position shown, with gradually increasing pressure to extend the range of the stretch. Many people may find this difficult initially and time and effort are needed to achieve the sort of levels shown by the illustration.

36a

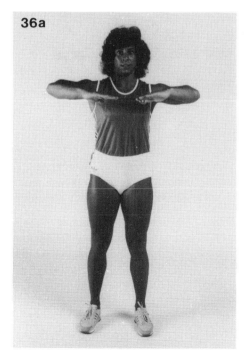

36b

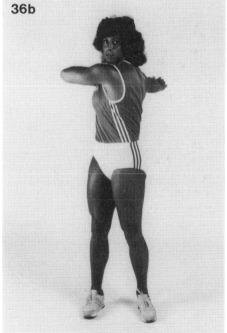

Exercise 37. Cat Stretch

Starting in the kneeling position the spine should first be arched fully upwards with the head being bent down between the arms. Next, with a gradual and controlled movement, extend the head upwards and let the spine sag downwards as far as it can go without undue pressure. Initially, the exercise should be done without forcing, but, as mobility improves, increased pressure may be used in each direction.

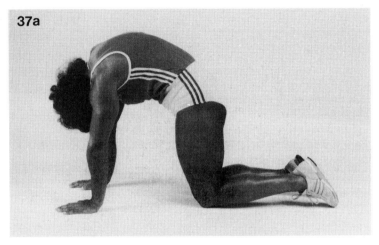

37a

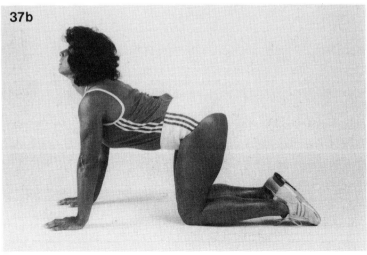

37b

Exercise 38. Forehead to Knee

Starting in the kneeling position, the head should be bent down between the arms at the same time as the knee is brought up towards the forehead. This should be done without creating any discomfort, but as far as can reasonably be achieved. The knee is then replaced beside the other one and the head stretched back to the straight position. This is then repeated with the alternate knee. In the early stages, there may be a large gap between the knee and the forehead, but, as the mobility of the spine increases, this gap should steadily diminish.

38 a

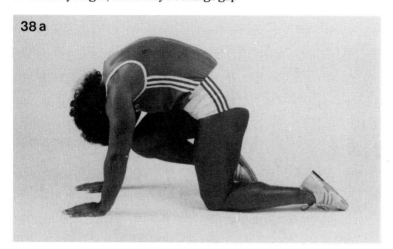

38 b

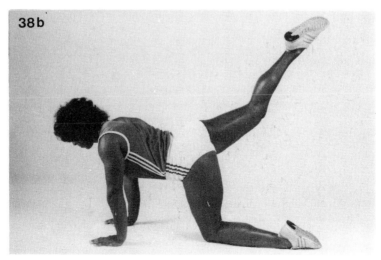

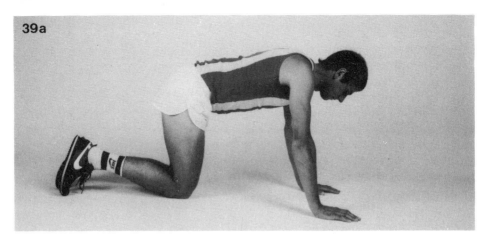

39a

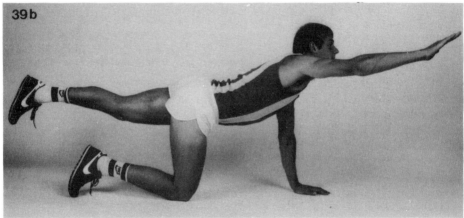

39b

Exercise 39.
Opposite Arm and Leg Stretch

Starting in the kneeling position, stretch out the left arm and the right leg and stretch the head and neck slightly upwards. Arms and legs are then returned to the commencement position and the process is repeated with the opposite arms and legs. As the body generally becomes fitter and stronger, the stretch position can be held for a longer period of time and a greater amount of stretch applied.

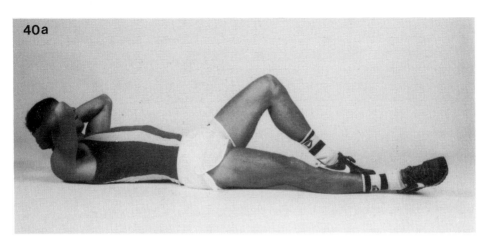

40a

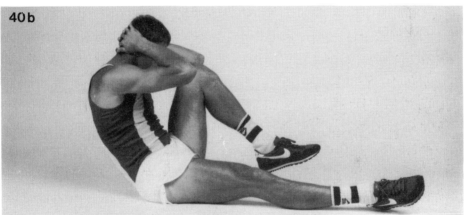

40b

Exercise 40.
Sit-ups to Alternate Knees

Lying on the back with the hands behind the neck, one knee is raised towards the mid point of the body, whilst the head and shoulders are lifted in a convergent direction. Once the maximum lift of both is achieved, return to the commencing position and repeat with the opposite knee. As strength and mobility increases, the gap between the knee and the head should diminish, the control of the exercise becomes better, and it should be possible to hold the position for longer.

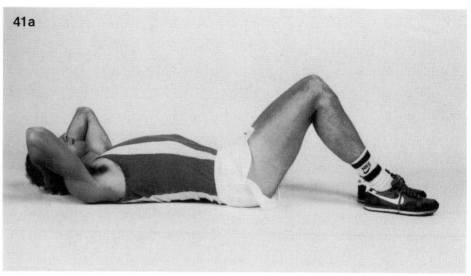

41a

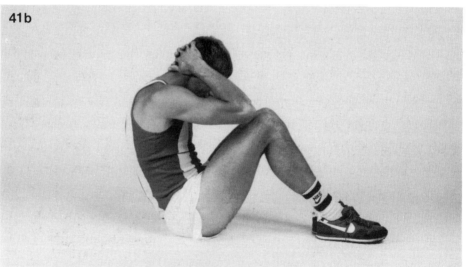

41b

Exercise 41. Sit-ups to Both Knees

With the knees bent and the hands behind
the neck as shown, curl up using the muscles
steadily rather than jerkily, and bring the
forehead up towards the knees. If a full lift
cannot be obtained initially, further
perseverance will gradually increase the
available movement.

42a

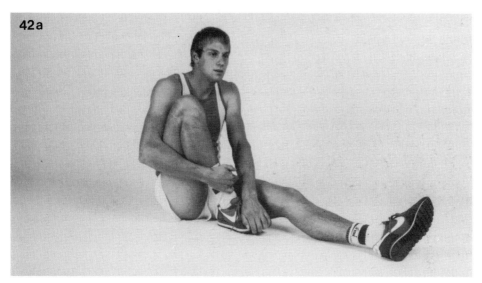

42b

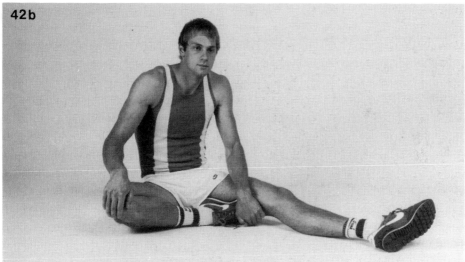

Exercise 42. Hip Stretch

Commence in the position illustrated and then stretch to the second position shown, gradually increasing pressure to extend the range of the stretch. Many people may find this difficult initially and time and effort are needed to achieve the sort of levels shown by the illustration.

Exercise 43. Kneeling Press-ups

Commence in a kneeling position with the back straight. The arms should then be bent until the face is lowered to the floor, and then straightened again to raise the body back to the original position. It is important to make sure that the legs stay still throughout this movement as it is designed to increase mobility around the hips.

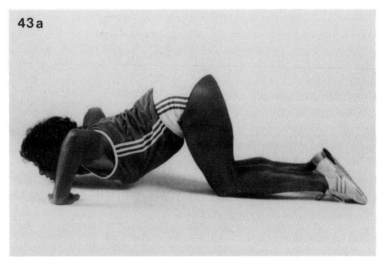

43 a

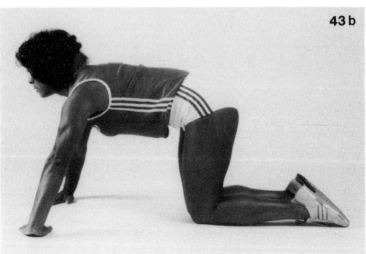

43 b

Exercise 44. Sitting Leg Stretch

This exercise can be done either with two chairs as in the illustration, or using a bench in similar fashion. Get comfortable prior to commencing the stretch and then gradually increase the amount of the stretch as the body loosens up under pressure. This exercise should never be forced, but rather relaxed into until a good degree of movement is obtained, whereupon some pressure may be added to increase the overall mobility. As it becomes easier to reach down the leg in the stretch, further pressure can be added steadily to even further increase the joints' range of movement.

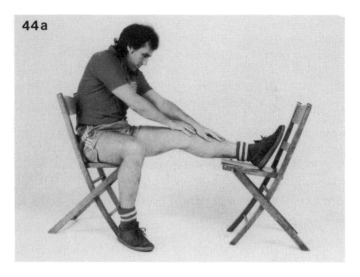

44a

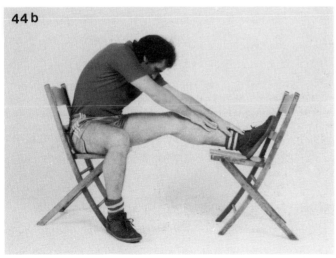

44b

Exercise 45.
Touching Alternate Feet

Commence in the starting position illustrated and then, bending forward, rotate the body to touch the right foot with the left hand. Repeat the movement, touching the left foot with the right hand. Make sure that the body describes as big a circle as possible and always keep the knees slightly bent.

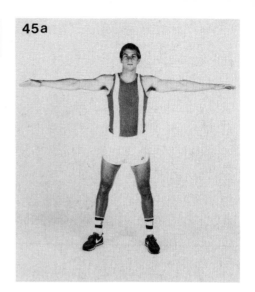

45a

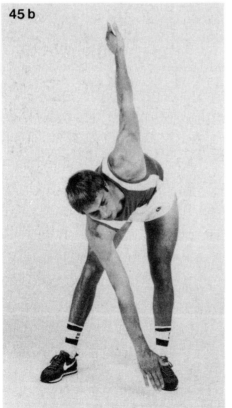

45b

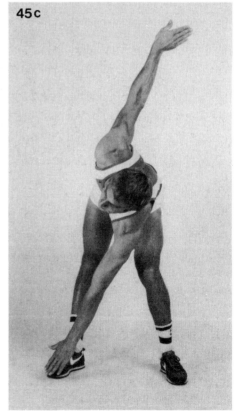

45c

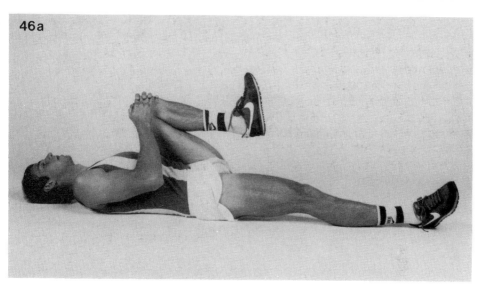

46 a

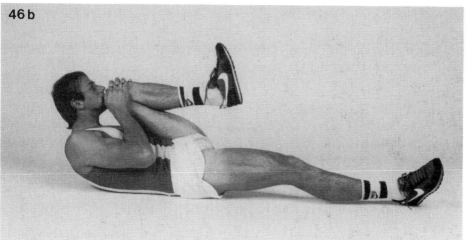

46 b

Exercise 46. Knee Clasp

Starting in the position illustrated, bring the knee towards the chest and then apply steady pressure with the hands to increase the range of stretch achieved. As mobility improves, the knee will come closer and tighter to the chest, and a greater awareness of low back stretching will be achieved. The exercise is repeated with alternate knees.

Exercise 47. Double Player Sit

It is important to make sure that the feet are well placed prior to undertaking this exercise, as slipping or sliding can cause problems. Both players should be firmly interlocked and lower slowly down to the right angled position as in the illustration, hold this for a count of 15 and then slowly back up.

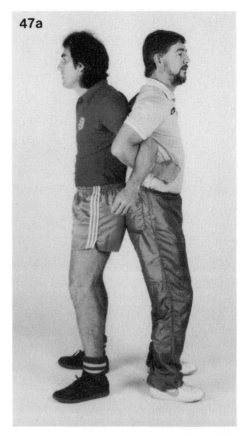

47a

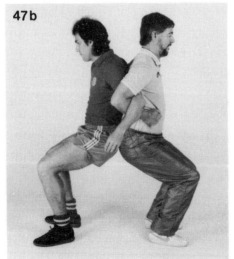

47b

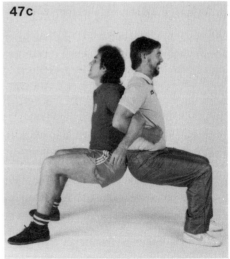

47c

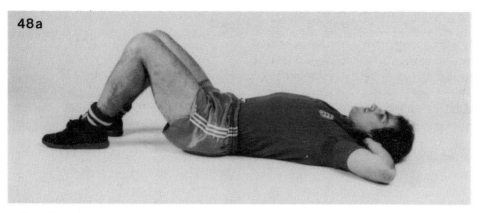

48a

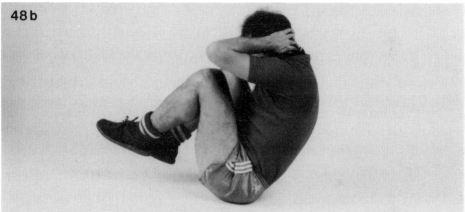

48b

Exercise 48. Figure of 'U' Sit-up

In this exercise, raise the feet and the head simultaneously from the starting position shown to try to achieve as near as possible the illustrated finishing position. In the early stages it may be very difficult, but as the muscles improve and the mobility increases, it will become easier to achieve the exercise in total. The stronger one becomes, the more controlled the movement will be and the final position may be held for a second or two before lowering back to recommence.

Exercise 49. Abdominal Press

Lie on the back with knees bent and feet flat on the ground. Then exhale and flatten the whole spine as much as possible against the floor. Hold this flattened position for 10 seconds and then relax and allow the spine to come away from the floor.

49a

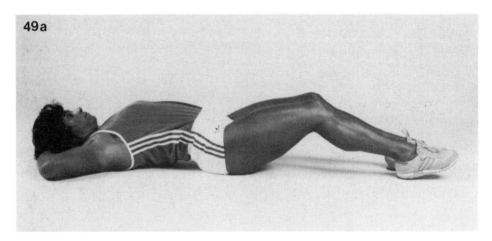

49b

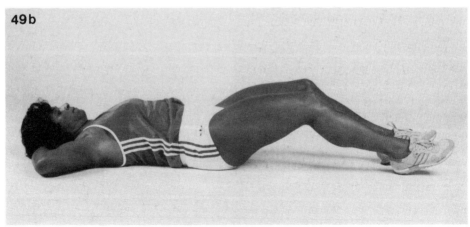

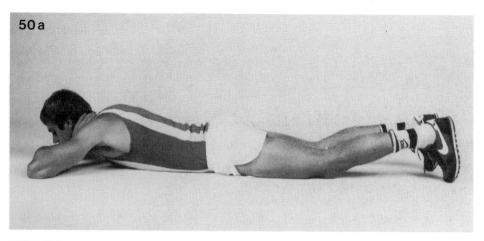

50 a

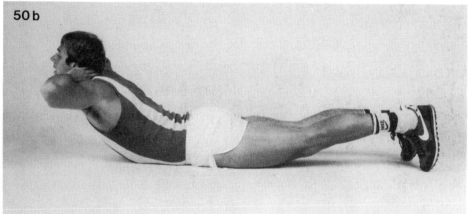

50 b

Exercise 50. Chest Raises

Lie down flat with the hands clasped behind the neck and relaxed, then raise the whole upper trunk, bringing the elbows up, raising the head and neck backwards and creating as much of an arch as is possible. Hold the position for a moment and then relax to the commencing position. As body tone improves, this exercise may be forced further and further, and the position may be held for a longer period of time.

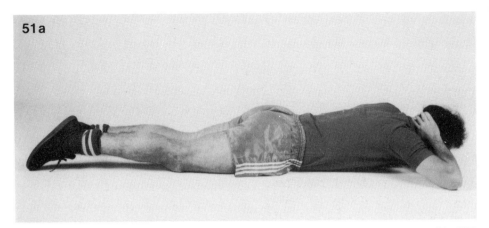

51a

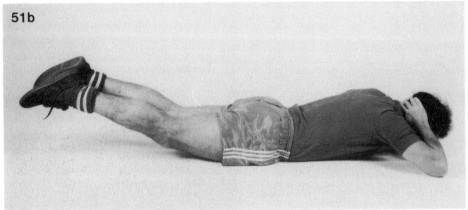

51b

Exercise 51. Leg Lifts

Commence lying face down with hands behind the neck and elbows resting on the floor. Raise the legs upwards as far as is possible without lifting the upper trunk. After holding the maximum lift for a few moments, lower the legs back to the commencing position, relax briefly and then repeat. As exercise improves the tone and mobility of the body, the leg lift will become higher and the position may be held for longer. It is possible, initially, that virtually no lift will be achieved, but perseverance will gradually increase this until the exercise can be done correctly.

Exercise 52. Salmon Raise

Lie face down with hands clasped behind the neck and elbows resting on the floor to commence. Then raise the feet off the ground and arch the head upwards, forcing back the elbows and raising the upper body at the same time. The resultant position should be an arc, which can gradually be increased as body mobility and strength develops. The position may be held for longer and longer as muscle power dictates.

52a

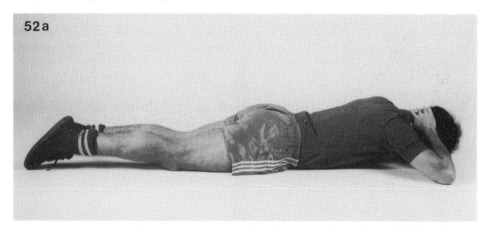

52b

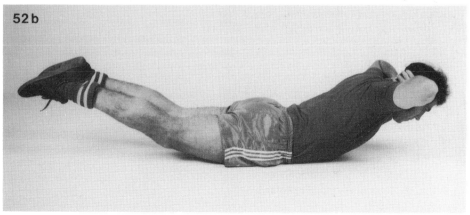

53a

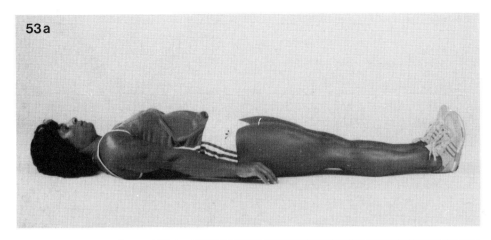

53b

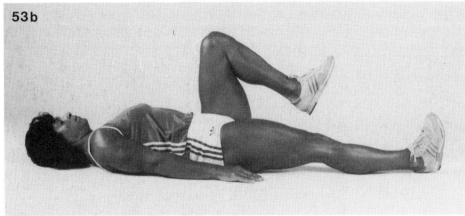

Exercise 53. Alternate Knee Raises

Lying on the back with the legs straight, first one knee and then the other is brought up towards the chest, then returned to its original position.

Exercise 54. One-handed Press-ups

Initially, this exercise, primarily for racquet sports, will be very difficult to do, but even to attempt it will fulfil the necessary requirements until sufficient strength is obtained in the non-playing arm to allow the exercise to be more fully completed.

Exercise 55. Press Ups

Supporting the weight of the body on the arms and pushing upwards until the arms are fully extended, it is important to ensure that the back stays straight and that the movement is slow and controlled. If the exercise is rushed, much of the benefit is lost.

55

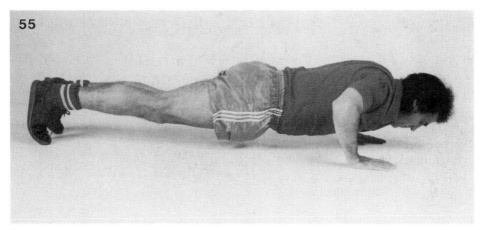

56

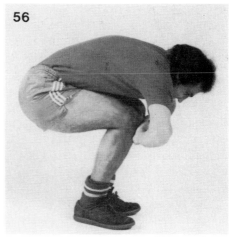

Exercise 56. Squatting

This is a matter of coming down to get the backside as close to the heels as possible, whilst keeping the feet flat on the floor. When maximum stretch is reached, straighten up and repeat the movement at a controlled but reasonable pace.

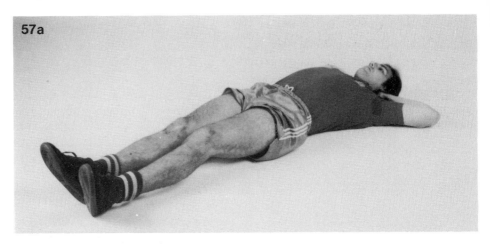

57a

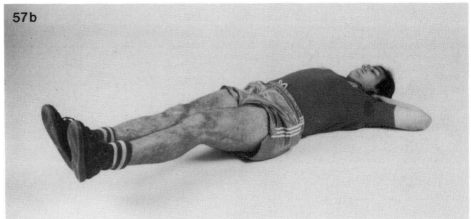

57b

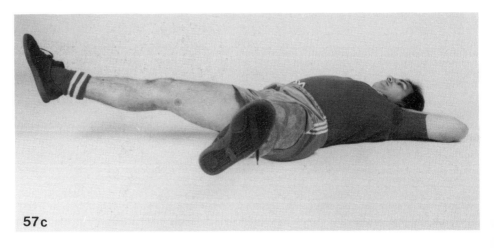

57c

Exercise 57.
Leg Raise 9 in, Open & Close

As can be seen from the illustration, the feet are raised 9 in from the floor with the head flat on the ground. The legs are then opened and closed slowly and steadily 5 times before the feet are lowered to the ground.

Exercise 58. Squat Thrusts

It is important in this exercise to make sure that the knees come right up (as shown) and that subsequently the leg is fully straightened in a piston fashion. As strength increases and mobility becomes greater, the speed and force of the exercise should be steadily increased. The exercise is not effective unless the full range of movement is carried out.

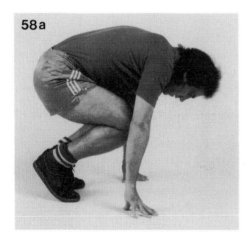

58a

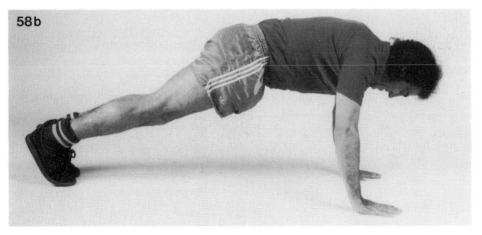

58b

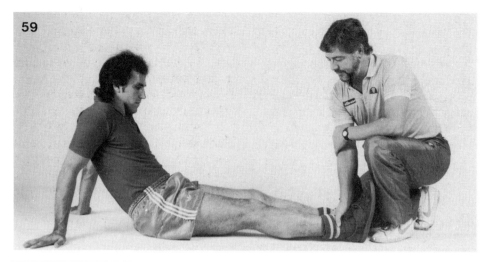

59

Exercise 59.
Ankle Restrained Leg Lift

Commence as illustrated with leg straight and ankle firmly held to the ground. With knee locked, push as hard as possible to attempt to raise the foot from the ground, and maintain the effort for a count of 3 and then relax. This exercise should be repeated until the muscle feels thoroughly tired, and as strength increases, with ever greater effort to lift.

Exercise 60
Double Ankle Restrained Leg Lift

The same position as in the previous exercise, but with both legs fixed. Ensure that the movement is slow and controlled. If the exercise is rushed, much of the benefit is lost.

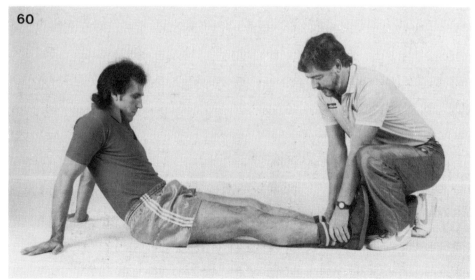

60

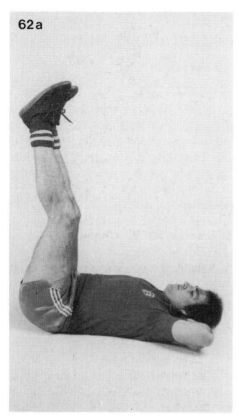

62a

Exercise 61. Single Knee Squat

With the back straight and feet together, stand by a chair which can be used for support, and raise one foot from the ground. Without tilting forward, slowly bend the knee until lowered as far as is comfortably possible, count to three and then slowly straighten out. This should be repeated until the leg feels really tired, and then undertaken on the opposite leg. As muscle strength increases, it will be possible to go both lower and more slowly.

Exercise 62. Straight Leg Lowering

Commence in the position shown, with the legs at right angles to the thighs, then lower them slowly down to a 45° angle. Count slowly to 3 before returning the legs to the commencing position. This should be repeated 3 times and then the legs may drop down to relax and thereby complete the exercise.

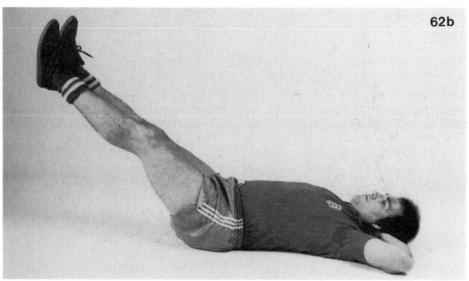

62b

10. CYCLING

Cycling, as a hobby and a sport, is becoming ever more popular and all forms are getting much greater television coverage than used to be the case in the past. Modern technology has developed very lightweight and sophisticated bicycles and, as with all sports, the physical efforts and pressures of being competitive are ever greater. Whether cycling for pleasure or competition, it is important to follow all the basic recommendations outlined earlier in the book and to achieve a very good level of basic fitness to produce the necessary stamina and strength.

Apart from basic fitness, the bulk of cycling training is, of necessity, done on a bicycle and, therefore, it is important to make sure that regular riding is undertaken, as well as very specific training for specific events. The main sources of problems for cyclists are in the knees, ankles and, particularly, the low back. The latter undergoes considerable strain because of the angle at which the spine is bent, coupled to the amount of force thrusting through the hips whilst pedalling. There is no doubt from a postural point of view that the old and 'Aunt Sally'-style upright bicycle put far less stress upon the spinal structures. The unnatural curvature induced by a modern competition bicycle tends to take the pelvis out of alignment, which then means that the knees and ankles cannot function through their normal range and therefore become prone to problems. In order to prevent the steady onset of actual or potential leg damage, it is important to do the following spinal mobilization exercises immediately before and, particularly, after any riding has taken place.

Apart from the above exercises, it is particularly pertinent to cyclists to remember the old adage to stand tall, walk tall and sit tall. The various forces applied to the spine whilst cycling tend to pressurize it and close the gaps between the individual vertebrae, and this can cause problems unless compensatory effort is made. One should always get the feel of stretching up away from the feet and practise the postural advice given in the earlier section, 'Keeping your body in trim'.

Exercise routine
The following exercises are illustrated in the Centre Section.

(Exercise 37)
Cat stretch — repeat 10 times, building up to 20 times.
(Exercise 38)
Forehead to knee — commence with 10, build up to 20.
(Exercise 49)
Abdominal press — commence with 10, build up to 20.
(Exercise 51)
Leg lift — commence with 10, build up to 20.
(Exercise 50)
Chest raise — commence with 10, build up to 20.
(Exercise 49)
Abdominal press — repeat 10 times.
(Exercise 52)
Salmon raise — commence with 10, build up to 20.
(Exercise 3)
Trunk twisting — repeat 10 times each way.

(Exercise 1)
Hip rotation — repeat 10 times each way.
(Exercise 39)
Opposite arm and leg stretch — repeat 10 times each way.
(Exercise 37)
Cat stretch — repeat 15 times.
(Exercise 49)
Abdominal press — repeat 15 times.
(Exercise 40)
Sit-ups to alternate knees — repeat 10 times to each knee.
(Exercise 2)
Side stretching — repeat 5 times to each side.

(Exercise 9)
Alternate leg stretch — repeat 5 times each way.
(Exercise 1)
Hip rotation — repeat 5 times each way.
(Exercise 52)
Salmon raise — repeat 10 times.
(Exercise 49)
Abdominal press — repeat 10 times.
(Exercise 37)
Cat stretch — repeat 15 times.

11. SWIMMING AND BOARDSAILING

Swimming both competitively and purely for pleasure has, in recent years, increased greatly in popularity, partly due to the greater availability of modern and pleasant swimming pools. Boardsailing, or windsurfing as it is frequently called, is a modern sport but in order to pursue it a good swimming capability is really an essential. From the point of view of training and fitness, both require the same fundamental pattern, with boardsailing having a few extra requirements in relation to back exercise which can very logically follow on. Hence the two sports can be dealt with in the same chapter.

Taken gently, and not on a competitive basis, swimming is a very beneficial exercise for the body and, indeed, is used remedially by many enlightened practitioners for their patients. Because the upward force of buoyancy exerted by the water helps, in effect, to reduce gravitational pressure on the body, joints can move more freely and follow greater arcs of range without causing as many stresses as is normally the case. From the point of view of sport, however, the amount of stress applied in the course of the activity is very much greater and, therefore, it is important to make sure that one is adequately prepared to be able to push the body physically hard without causing problems.

The neck and the low back are the two areas which come under the greatest strain in the course of swimming, and the low back particularly in the process of diving. In diving, when part of the body is in the water, the part which is outside can have a powerful lever effect on that which has entered the water. It is important that one should learn to dive properly in order to minimize one of the main potential sources of back injuries.

The normal fitness advice given in the early chapters of the book should, of course, be followed as a basis for specialization, and the exercises outlined below should be used as a warm-up routine prior to commencing to swim. After a long and hard swim or a very competitive one, they should also be used as a cool-down routine to prevent any tension or stiffness building up in the body prior to further exercise.

Warm up/cool down exercises
(Illustrated in Centre Section)

(Exercise 37)
Cat stretch — commence with 5, build up to 20.
(Exercise 38)
Forehead to knee — commence with 5 each side, build up to 20.
(Exercise 39)
Opposite arm and leg stretch — commence with 10, build up to 20.
(Exercise 46)
Knee clasp — commence with 5, build up to 15.
(Exercise 9)
Alternate leg stretch — repeat 5 times each way.
(Exercise 4)
Hands between legs — repeat 5 times.

(Exercise 41)
Sit-ups to both knees — commence with 5, build up to 20.

Presuming that one has followed the basic advice and used the warm-up routine described above, for boardsailing the following exercises should be practised twice a day, for at least a month before the season starts, as well as on a regular basis during the actual boardsailing season.

Training exercises
(Illustrated in Centre Section)

(Exercise 52)
Salmon raise — commence with 5, build up to 20.
(Exercise 49)
Abdominal press — commence with 10, build up to 20.
(Exercise 37)
Cat stretch — repeat 10 times.
(Exercise 4)
Hands between legs — repeat 10 times.
(Exercise 3)
Trunk twisting — repeat 5 times each way.
(Exercise 1)
Hip rotation — repeat five times each way.
(Exercise 37)
Cat stretch — repeat 10 times.
(Exercise 1)
Hip rotation — repeat 10 times each way.
(Exercise 3)
Trunk twisting — repeat 10 times.
(Exercise 49)
Abdominal press — repeat 10 times.
(Exercise 40)
Sit-ups to alternate knees — repeat 10 times each way.
(Exercise 52)
Salmon raise — repeat 10 times each way.

(Exercise 57)
Leg raise 9 in, open and close — commence with 5, build up to 25.
(Exercise 51)
Leg lifts — commence with 10, build up to 20.
(Exercise 50)
Chest raises — commence with 10, build up to 20.
(Exercise 57)
Leg raise 9 in, open and close — commence with 5, build up to 20.
(Exercise 20)
Squatting star jumps — commence with 10, build up to 20.
(Exercise 48)
Figure 'U' sit-ups — commence with 5, build up to 20.
(Exercise 55)
Press ups — commence with 10, build up to 20.
(Exercise 62)
Straight leg lowering — commence with 5, build up to 15.
(Exercise 37)
Cat stretch — repeat 10 times.
(Exercise 2)
Side stretching — repeat 10 times each way.
(Exercise 4)
Hands between legs — repeat 10 times.

As can be seen, a lot of emphasis is placed on low back strengthening, and the associated strengthening of the abdominal muscles, so that no damage is suffered whilst pulling the sail out of the water, which is the most traumatic part of the sport. The more skilled one becomes at boardsailing, the less one has to undertake this heaving process, but at this stage the strength and mobility of the back enables one to sail for longer with less after-effect and to a greater capability.

12. WATER SKIING

Whilst water skiing has become very much more popular as a holiday occupation over the last few years, it is only very recently that there has been a major increase in public interest and involvement in it as an all-year-round activity. In this country, of course, it is much more difficult to pursue because of the weather, but wetsuits and hardy people make it possible for the bulk of the time. Water skiing is, of course, a sport that can involve quite a high degree of traumatic injury, from simple first-aid problems such as rope burns to very much more major damage to the arms, legs or spine due to falls and accidents, particularly in relation to jumping.

Because both the upper and lower body need to be in good physical condition to perform effectively, it is very important to take adequate time preparing to undertake water skiing as a sport. For those who ski regularly, the routine suggested below should be followed for one month before the season starts, whilst for those who ski only occasionally — ie, on holiday — it should be followed for three-four weeks prior to going on holiday and undertaking the activity.

The exercises illustrated below should be followed as a daily routine, presuming that the advice given in the early chapters on basic health and fitness has already been put into action. The programme should be preceded by a short run, consisting of five minutes jogging, five minutes running, five minutes hard running, and five minutes jogging. At the completion of the run, jog gently on the spot until pulse and heart rate settles down to near normal, then commence the exercise programme outlined below.

Exercise programme

The following exercises are illustrated in the Centre Section.

(Exercise 37)
Cat stretch — commence with 5, build up to 10.
(Exercise 38)
Forehead to knee — commence with 5, build up to 10.
(Exercise 49)
Abdominal press — commence with 10, build up to 20.
(Exercise 55)
Press ups — commence with 5 build up to 20.
(Exercise 58)
Squat thrusts — commence with 10, build up to 30.
(Exercise 50)
Chest raise — commence with 10, build up to 30.
(Exercise 57)
Leg raise 9 in, open and close — commence with 5, build up to 20.
(Exercise 41)
Sit-ups to both knees — commence with 10, build up to 20.
(Exercise 58)
Squat thrusts — commence with 10 times, build up to 20.
(Exercise 20)
Squatting star jumps — commence with 10, build up to 20.
(Exercise 49)
Abdominal press — repeat 10 times.

(Exercise 40)
Sit-ups to alternate knees — commence with 10, build up to 20.
(Exercise 41)
Sit-ups to both knees — commence with 10, build up to 20.
(Exercise 37)
Cat stretch — repeat 10 times.
(Exercise 1)
Hip rotation — repeat 5 times each way.
(Exercise 3)
Trunk twisting — repeat 5 times each way.
(Exercise 4)
Hands between legs — repeat 10 times.

The exercises recommended are particularly designed to improve low back mobility and strength, knee mobility and strength, and neck and shoulder mobility. These factors are essential if unnecessary injury is to be avoided. Unless the joints are flexible and mobile as well as strong, strains and muscle pulls are almost inevitable.

During the season, or perhaps whilst on holiday, the shorter programme outlined below should be followed, in order to maintain mobility and reduce injury potential.

(Exercise 37)
Cat stretch — repeat 10 times.
(Exercise 38)
Forehead to knee — repeat 10 times.
(Exercise 49)
Abdominal press — repeat 20 times.
(Exercise 58)
Squat thrusts — repeat 20 times.
(Exercise 41)
Sit-ups to both knees — repeat 10 times.
(Exercise 3)
Trunk twisting — repeat 10 times.
(Exercise 4)
Hands between legs — repeat 10 times.

Because of the power applied to the body, water skiing is a sport that should not be undertaken unless feeling fit and well and, if in any doubt, sensible professional advice should be sought.

13. SKIING

Because of the dramatic improvement in transport and communications, skiing, which was once the preserve of the wealthy, is now available to almost everybody and, indeed, most secondary schools offer skiing trips for their pupils at some stage. It is a very stimulating and exhilarating sport, but also a very physically demanding one and the potential danger areas of undertaking skiing without proper training are many. A high level of physical stamina is required if one is to be able to continue to ski for a period of hours without becoming sufficiently tired to make mistakes. Tiredness almost invariably leads to error, and skiing in a tired error-prone state can very easily result in broken bones, damaged joints and sometimes even worse.

Presuming that anybody who wishes to go skiing has followed the basic concepts of general fitness laid out in the early chapters of this book, then there is still specific preparation necessary prior to departure and certain routines should be used during the course of the skiing holiday.

In order to be able to ski effectively, the knees must be both strong and mobile. Without these two factors, good skiing is almost impossible, so a series of knee exercises such as those laid out below should be done three times a day for at least one month prior to going on holiday. These exercises should also be repeated first thing in the morning before beginning the day's sport.

Knee exercises
(Illustrated in Centre Section)

(Exercise 55)
Squatting — repeat 10 times.
(Exercise 46)
Knee clasp — commence with 5, build up to 15.
(Exercise 32)
Knee exercising — commence with 10 to each leg, build up to 20.
(Exercise 60)
Single knee squat — repeat until the leg feels tired (described but not illustrated).
(Exercise 55)
Squatting — repeat 15 times, slowly.
(Exercise 20)
Squatting star jumps — commence with 5, build up to 20.
(Exercise 57)
Squat thrusts — commence with 5, build up to 20.

Another area of the body that takes considerable strain during skiing is the low back, and this should also be exercised and strengthened for at least a month, and again warmed up each day before taking to the slopes. A series of back mobilizing and strengthening exercises is outlined below and if these and the knee exercises are done regularly, then maximum pleasure can be achieved during the course of the holiday.

Back mobilizing and strengthening exercises (Illustrated in Centre Section)

(Exercise 37)
Cat stretch — repeat 10 times.
(Exercise 38)
Forehead to knee — repeat 10 times.

(Exercise 50)
Chest raise — repeat 10 times.
(Exercise 51)
Leg lift — repeat 10 times.
(Exercise 52)
Salmon raise — repeat 10 times.
(Exercise 55)
Press ups — repeat 10 times.
(Exercise 40)
Sit-ups to alternate knees — repeat 10 times
    each way.
(Exercise 41)
Sit-ups to both knees — repeat 15 times.
(Exercise 49)
Abdominal press — repeat 10 times.
(Exercise 46)
Knee clasp — commence with 5, build up
    to 15.

Skiing entails a fairly high risk of traumatic injury, as falls can frequently lead to breaks, fractures, and serious sprains, to say nothing of ligamentous damage. If any accident takes place and anything other than bad bruising appears to be the problem, it is most important to have expert medical attention as soon as is possible. Many injuries will only be short-term, so long as they are treated correctly and rapidly, but if left they can become major and long-term interferences with function. Nearly all ski resorts now have well-equipped medical centres with staff who are thoroughly used to the type of accidental damage which can occur during a fall or crash. If injuries have been sustained in previous skiing trips, then it is doubly important to make sure that the areas which have been affected, especially if it be the back or the knees, are well exercised and strengthened prior to the next attempt.

It is wise to undertake a programme of regular running for some time prior to a skiing trip, unless regular sport of some other type is played, giving the necessary stamina levels to be able to ski throughout the course of the day.

14. ROWING

Rowing is a particularly demanding sport physically, in as much as one is intending to move a reasonably heavy object by sheer physical power alone. One only has to watch closely the strain and tension on the faces of top rowers to realize just how much is being put into the function of rowing or sculling.

Far and away the single most common injury to rowers is low back trouble, both during their career and, in many cases, soon after retiring from the sport. In most cases, this is because of ill preparation and because coaching techniques tend to concentrate on the basic skills of rowing rather than maintaining the necessary spinal alignment to prevent any impairment of function.

Because of the strength and stamina requirements, it is important to follow the basic advice given in the early chapters on producing healthy and effective tissue, and of course all the exercise and postural advice should be followed energetically. On top of this, and particularly in the pre-competition season, the following series of exercises should be done twice a day. During the competition season, once a day should be satisfactory.

If the exercises, whose purpose is to not only improve the strength of the postural muscles and the low back but above all to increase the mobility of the back and its associated joints, are practised regularly, this will help to offset the effects of the heavy forces applied to the lower back. Immediately prior to warming up in the boat, and immediately after leaving the boat, it is very important to undertake a series of stretching exercises to make sure that no lasting stiffnesses are left to cause problems as they accumulate. The following series of exercises are not very time-consuming but may well be the stitch which saves nine as far as the low back and the legs are concerned.

If any injury is sustained during the course of rowing, rapid and efficient attention should be sought, since to continue to row with problems can result in very much greater long-term ones resulting. An osteopath, chiropractor or a physiotherapist should be contacted as soon as possible to deal with any muscular or structural abnormalities which may have occurred as a result of intensive effort. A golden rule is always to resist the urge to row unless one really does feel in suitable, physical shape. Much damage is done by ill-founded beliefs that to carry on and 'work through it' will sort the problem out. When not actively involved in rowing, running is a good exercise to undertake, so long as it is done in proper shoes (preferably with air soles) and fast enough and for long enough to help improve general bodily stamina. A run of twenty minutes, with the first and last five minutes at a steadier pace, and the middle ten minutes at a rapid pace, is an ideal minimum, with the back stretching training exercises outlined here being undertaken before and after the run. All running and training should be followed by a warm shower, not much above body heat, and wherever available a short, sharp cold shower to finish off with. This should not be taken until the pulse rate has dropped to near normal and breathing has settled down.

Training exercises
(Illustrated in Centre Section)

(Exercise 37)
Cat stretch — commence with 5, build up to 20.
(Exercise 38)
Forehead to knee — commence with 5 each side, build up to 10.
(Exercise 1)
Hip rotation — repeat 5 times each way.
(Exercise 3)
Trunk twisting — repeat 5 times each way.
(Exercise 2)
Side stretching — repeat 10 times each way.
(Exercise 49)
Abdominal press — repeat 10 times.
(Exercise 50)
Chest raises — commence with 10, build up to 30.
(Exercise 51)
Leg lift — commence with 10, build up to 30.

(Exercise 49)
Abdominal press — repeat 15 times.
(Exercise 52)
Salmon raise — commence with 10, build up to 30.
(Exercise 40)
Sit-ups to alternate knees — commence with 5, build up to 20.
(Exercise 41)
Sit-ups to both knees — commence with 10, build up to 30.
(Exercise 49)
Abdominal press — repeat 10 times.
(Exercise 53)
Alternate knee raise — repeat 5 times for each knee.
(Exercise 37)
Cat stretch — repeat 10 times.
(Exercise 1)
Hip rotation — repeat 10 times each way.
(Exercise 4)
Hands between legs — repeat 10 times.

15. GOLF

There are many people who look upon golf as 'an old man's sport' but it is, in reality, a very physically and mentally demanding game. Its one great advantage is that it can be played by people of all ages on a genuinely competitive basis as it lends itself to a workable handicap system.

As a game, it causes a number of problems physically and golfers suffer a wide selection of injuries which are, of necessity, almost totally self-inflicted. Unlike physically competitive games and contact sports, one is not knocked, jostled or hit by the opposing player, so the sort of problems suffered are due either to poor technique, or an inadequately fit and mobile body or a combination of both. Because of the nature of a golf swing, there are a number of conflicting stresses placed upon the body. The rotation of the shoulders around the head is of an entirely different nature from the movement of the hips which is going on at the same time as the upper body movement. One of the main problem areas for golfers is the low back because of this complicated turn and thrust movement. The less smooth the basic swing, and the harder one tries to hit the ball, then the greater the amount of stress which is applied to the low back and hips during the execution of the shot.

Whilst in no way attempting to give coaching or lessons in golf, it is important from the body's point of view not to try to over-swing or use excessive muscular effort, thus creating undue pressures for the body to absorb. The art of hitting a golf ball a long way is dependent upon smoothness and timing, and these factors help greatly in reducing injury potential.

Many club golfers will dash straight from a twenty or thirty minute drive in a car, into the clubhouse for a quick change, grab a trolley, rush to the first tee and strike the ball hopefully down the fairway. From the body's point of view, this is a disastrous process since none of the muscles required for the golf swing have had any loosening or warming prior to that first moment of impact on the tee. Before any game of golf, even before hitting balls on the practice green, a simple series of exercises to loosen the back and the arms and get blood flowing in the appropriate muscles should be undertaken as outlined below and illustrated in the Centre Section.

Warm up exercises
(Illustrated in Centre Section)

(Exercise 36)
Hip swing — repeat 5 times each way.
(Exercise 1)
Hip rotation — repeat 5 times each way.
(Exercise 2)
Side stretching — commence with 5 each way, build up to 10.
(Exercise 11)
Neck stretch — repeat 5 times each way.
(Exercise 33)
Shoulder swing — commence with 5, build up to 10.
(Exercise 24)
Double arm swing — commence with 5, build up to 20.

(Exercise 34)

Back turn using golf club — repeat 8 times each way.

(Exercise 35)

Swing and turn using golf club — commence with 5 each way, build up to 15.

One of the long-term dangers of golf is that it is both a one-sided and lop-sided game. If you look at somebody in position for a golf swing, then you can see the imbalance created in the proper stance. To make sure that the pursuit of pleasure on a golf course does not cause day-to-day problems, it is important to compensate for the one-sidedness of the game. This is quite easily done in the game of golf by spending five minutes or so at the end of a match swinging a club in the reverse fashion, leading with the left hand and doing the reverse activity, and just swinging to and fro so that the complete opposite set of muscles follow the same pattern and usage as those of the other side. If this is made a regular part of one's playing habits, then it can save a tremendous amount of problems as time passes by.

Hand and wrist problems and 'golfer's elbow' are other sources of discomfort, aggravation, and interference with the ability to play the game. In most cases, this is due to two factors: one is gripping the clubs excessively tightly with the whole arm rather than just the hand — which means that the wrist and elbow joints are under pressure when striking the ball, and secondly, in many cases, from sheer lack of muscle tone in the wrist and forearm. Another source of these problems is hitting the ground hard on a number of occasions and the resultant shock. To reduce the chance of this happening, either a small wrist exerciser should be used or an old tennis ball which has gone a little soft should be held in the palm of the hand and squeezed into with the fingers. Whilst doing these exercises, rotate the wrists and move the arms round to different angles to maintain full mobility whilst increasing the strength.

If damage does result from impact and the wrist or elbow is painful, one of the most effective treatments for this condition is alternate hot and cold bathing, using two bowls of water, one as hot as the elbow or wrist can comfortably be placed into and the other as cold as it runs from the tap. Where possible, put a large handful of epsom salts in the hot water and then bathe the affected area for three minutes in the hot and one minute in the cold, repeating this process so that eight minutes treatment are used in all. This should be done at least twice a day and, where possible, three times. It is also important to rest the affected area until the pain is dramatically reduced, as otherwise it tends to recur very quickly.

It should be remembered that the average golf course is four to five miles in length and, therefore, if one only plays on a once per week basis, the very least preparation that should be taken during the week is to consistently walk some two to three miles per day which will not only reduce the chance of damaging legs, ankles, knees etc, but will improve one's game, as a solid platform for the swing is a critical part of the game itself.

16. TABLE TENNIS

Table tennis is a sport with a huge following throughout the world, particularly, of course, in countries such as China where it is the national sport, and in any areas where space restricts outside sports.

The modern game has increased dramatically in speed and skill requirements and, as with nearly all events, the quality of the equipment has necessitated greater fitness and ability on the player's part. Table tennis is certainly not a gentle game of pit-pat, and at any serious level the game of 'ping pong' has died a death.

The modern game requires a high level of mobility and the ability to move rapidly in any direction whilst maintaining a balanced platform from which to play a variety of shots. Add onto this the need to turn the bat to use the appropriate face for whatever shot is to be undertaken and it is quite clear why the fitness and mobility side of the game must be taken for granted if the mind and hands are to perform their necessary tasks without restriction.

Once the basic fitness recommendations have been followed, then players are ready to raise their level of physical preparation to a point ready for the table tennis coach's skills. A sensible run should be undertaken each day with a warm up and a cool down routine of exercises (as outlined below) being used before and after the run. The run should last for about twenty minutes, with the first five minutes being taken at a steady jog, the next ten minutes at a good pace, and the last five minutes at a steady jog prior to returning to base for the exercises. The same programme of exercises should be used as a back loosening and mobilizing routine before any game, and between games if any period of wait is involved.

Warm up/cool down exercises
(Illustrated in Centre Section)

(Exercise 3)
Trunk twisting — repeat 10 times.
(Exercise 1)
Hip rotation — repeat 10 times.
(Exercise 2)
Side stretching — repeat 5 times.
(Exercise 9)
Alternate leg stretch — repeat 5 times each way.
(Exercise 37)
Cat stretch — commence with 10, build up to 20.
(Exercise 39)
Opposite arm and leg stretch — commence with 5, build up to 20.
(Exercise 38)
Forehead to knee — commence with 5, build up to 15.
(Exercise 4)
Hands between legs — repeat 10 times.

On the days when the run is not undertaken, the following fitness programme should be used, and for those who wish to pursue the game at the highest level, it should be done as a daily routine. The second exercise programme (outlined below) should be used to start off the training session.

Start of training session exercises
(Illustrated in Centre Section)

(Exercise 4)
Hands between legs — repeat 10 times.
(Exercise 38)
Forehead to knee — repeat 10 times.
(Exercise 46)
Knee clasp — repeat 5 times each way.
(Exercise 53)
Alternate knee raises — repeat 10 times each.

These basic exercises should then be followed by jogging on the spot for thirty seconds and running on the spot for thirty seconds, and repeated. The second session of the basic exercises should be followed by twenty squat thrusts, ten press-ups, ten salmon raises, twenty knees to the chest, ten squatting star jumps and a good session of jogging. After the jog, a series of ten 25-metre shuttles should be undertaken, followed by a five minute steady run, and then a series of five 50-metre shuttles. This should then be followed by the series of exercises as laid out below:

Training session exercises
(Illustrated in Centre Section)

(Exercise 45)
Touching alternate feet — repeat 10 times to each foot.
(Exercise 4)
Hands between legs — repeat 10 times.
(Exercise 38)
Forehead to knee — repeat 10 times.
(Exercise 39)
Opposite arm and leg stretch — repeat 10 times to each side.
(Exercise 28)
Elbow stretch inhalation — repeat 5 times.

These exercises should be followed by another five-minute steady run and then

twenty 20-metre sprints flat out. This should be followed by two minutes jogging on the spot while the breathing settles down and the final series of exercises as laid out below should be followed by a gentle two-minute jog around to cool off prior to taking a blood heat shower and, where possible, a short, sharp, cold shower to finish with.

Table Tennis Fitness Programme Summary

Exercises
30 seconds jogging on the spot
30 seconds running on the spot
20 squat thrusts
10 press-ups
10 salmon raises
20 knees to chest
10 squatting star jumps
Jogging on the spot
10×25-metre shuttle sprints
5 minute run
5×50-metre shuttle sprints
5 minute run
20×20-metre flat out sprints
2 minutes jogging on the spot
Gentle 2 minutes jog around

Because of the nature of the sport, despite being one-sided, the amount of movement undertaken and body turning and rotation to a large degree is self-compensating. One does not get the tremendous variations in body size as with tennis, and the bulk of injury problems are in the shoulder, the low back or the knees, with the low back problem being the most prevalent. If a proper fitness programme, as outlined above, is undertaken then these areas of potential danger should be dramatically reduced, and above all one's standard of play should be considerably improved.

Where injury is sustained in the course of playing, it is very important to get early advice and treatment where necessary, particularly if the back is involved. For twists and sprains, simple home treatment for those is outlined in the final chapter, but for anything more serious, good professional advice should be taken as early as possible.

17. SPORTS INJURIES

There is much discussion in all branches of the medical world about sports medicine. There are many practitioners of orthodox medicine, physiotherapy, chiropractic and osteopathy who consider there is no such thing as sports medicine. They contend that any form of abnormality or injury is part of medicine itself and, therefore, should not be considered separately.

There is another school, however, of which the writer is a great protagonist, which considers that all people, either amateur or professional, undertaking sport need a very different approach as and when injury occurs. Professionally, advice is needed to improve the long-term career and, on an amateur basis, advice is helpful in relation to one's ability to maintain normal everyday life as well as undertake sport. The general medical approach of 'rest and wait and see' is not satisfactory for the person actively engaged in the pursuit of sport. Sports persons need to have: (a) a rapid and accurate diagnosis of their problem; (b) rapid and effective treatment of the injury subsequent to diagnosis; and (c) to be given an instant decision on whether or not they are fit to continue their chosen sport. If not, they need to know for how long they will be out of action. The absence of this information has, in many cases, resulted in apparently simple injuries becoming major injuries which can have a devastating effect on a sports person's professional career or an amateur's pleasure.

Alternative medicine, in the form of osteopathy, chiropractic and acupuncture, is having an ever-increasing impact on the world of sports injury treatment, and, in some countries, practitioners of one or other or a combination of the above skills are a regular part of the medical team of professional and amateur sports. In Britain we have been slow to appreciate the total importance of spinal and bony structure in the maintenance of fitness for sport but, of late, major progress has been made in this direction.

More and more general practitioners, orthopaedic surgeons and physiotherapists are not only becoming aware of and interested in sports medicine but are also beginning to co-operate with the alternative medicine practitioners with tremendous benefit to all those taking an active part in sport.

Sports injuries can be divided into two categories: traumatic and non-traumatic. Traumatic injuries are those induced by fall, impact, violent rotation or wrenching, or direct interference by outside forces. Non-traumatic injuries are pulls, strains and musculo-skeletal problems which occur during pursuit of a particular sport.

Although the two are separate entities, many traumatic injuries either occur because of, or are made worse because of, the basic unfitness of the person suffering the problem at the time. We will deal with traumatic injuries first.

The simplest kind of traumatic injuries are cuts, bruises and scratches or scrapes. It is important that every sports person or sporting club should have available simple, straight-forward first aid equipment such as antiseptic, lint, gauze, plaster and bandage, to deal with this type of problem. In physical contact sports where more serious injuries of this nature are possible, an adequately stocked first aid kit is essential and, wherever possible, somebody who knows how to use it.

Injuries, such as sprained ankles, twisted knees, sprained wrists and wrenched thumbs, are fairly commonplace in a number of sports. It is vital to know how to deal with these injuries correctly and they should be dealt with as follows. The first decision to make if the injury occurs during the course of a game is whether it is possible to play on, or whether one should immediately leave the field of play. If playing on, then it is always sensible to strap and support the damaged area, and ankle, wrist, Achilles, knee, and thumb strappings as illustrated on pages 121-127. Never rush the application of these strappings because, if they are to be effective, they need to be applied correctly. Improperly applied or ineffective strapping is, in many cases, more harmful than no strapping at all.

If it is decided to leave the field, or otherwise immediately after the game is over, the first application to any damaged area is that of ice. A supply should always be readily available at any sporting arena and this should be applied in a bag to the damaged area for a period of fifteen minutes. After this, particularly if there is any sign of heavy swelling, a strapping should be applied. This should be maintained in position for 24 hours, after which it should be removed and the damage reassessed. Where possible, professional advice should be given but, failing this, if the injury is still painful, alternate hot and cold bathing — that is, three minutes in water as hot as can be stood, and one minute in water as cold as available from the tap, repeated twice — should be applied at regular intervals. If swelling is still present at this point in time, a strong tubigrip or elastic support should be used in between bathing sessions. If a lot of pain is present in the joint, then a more firm strapping using *Elastoplast* should be applied as shown in the accompanying diagram.

Where heavy bruising is involved, an external application of tincture of arnica or witch hazel lotion on a pad of lint helps to reduce the amount of long-term damage. This should be applied over the site of the injury, fairly moist, left in place for a minimum of three-four hours and replaced if pain and discomfort is still present.

If at any time there is excessive pain or excessive swelling in any joint which has suffered damage, self-treatment should never be attempted and professional advice should be sought. If, during a game, a serious injury occurs — *particularly if the neck is involved* — *never move* the player until professional advice has been sought. Spinal damage, if badly handled, can lead to paralysis or worse, so always, *always*, if in doubt, wait! After injury, always exercise the affected joint back into action, and make sure it is fully functional before recommencing play. So many injuries recur and interfere with a player's ability for a whole season, purely and simply because playing has recommenced too soon. It is much better to be one week late playing than miss the rest of the season.

One should also remember that, after an injury, the leg or arm involved has usually lost a little of its muscle power and, if the injury has been prolonged, a considerable amount of strength has usually disappeared. To compensate for this, one should exercise either the arm or the leg or the wrist individually until one can visibly see that power has been restored and a balance regained.

Where broken limbs or dislocated joints are involved, professional help is obviously necessary, but steps should be taken to relieve the discomfort of the individual as soon and as much as is possible. Slings, inflatable splints, and a splittable stretcher should be available at every sports ground where contact sport takes place. The provision of these items of equipment could mean the difference between comfort or half an hour's agony for somebody who has suffered a serious injury. There is very little more painful than a broken bone or a dislocated joint, improperly stabilized whilst awaiting the trip to the hospital casualty department.

Every club or sporting group should attempt to ensure that it has available at any meeting or match at least one person who has a sound training in first aid and, better still, a good knowledge of sports medicine. The availability of such a person may, in extreme cases, save life, but in almost all cases will save pain and discomfort on the spot, and have a lasting effect on the remainder of the season. Doctors, osteopaths and physiotherapists are often only too pleased to become involved with sporting clubs, since they themselves are frequently engaged in the pursuit of some sport or other.

The non-traumatic injuries are suffered as a result of either inadequate preparation or some minor stiffness or tension which has gone undetected. Where muscles are pulled or torn, the immediate treatment is to apply ice which should be maintained on the site of the injury for fifteen minutes, following which a pressure bandage, a crepe bandage should be applied to the site of the injury. This helps to reduce or prevent the internal bleeding and will dramatically shorten the healing time of the injury. This pressure bandage should be maintained for 24 hours,

after which it should be tightened and maintained for another 24 hours. Thereafter, the injured site should be treated with alternate hot and cold bathing or spraying, either in a bowl or with a shower, dependent upon the position of the damage. This should be followed on a basis of three minutes hot and one minute cold, repeated twice. This should be done at least twice a day or, in the case of bad injuries, three or four times per day. As the pain decreases, then exercise and stretching of the area should be gradually increased, until such time as it feels normal.

Where an injury is regularly repeated, such as a torn ham-string or a groin strain, then professional advice should be sought as these are almost always due to some skeletal imbalance producing uneven muscle development and, therefore, vulnerability to over-reaching itself under strenuous activity.

In summary, to be able to deal with injuries as and when they occur as effectively as possible, the following procedure should be followed:

1. Establish communication with doctors, osteopaths, chiropractors, physiotherapists etc, who are available within the area with an interest in sports medicine.
2. Make sure that one of the above, and a skilled first aid person is available at any sporting meeting.
3. Make sure that adequate first aid supplies are always maintained, that their position is known, and that they are readily accessible.
4. In contact sports, make sure that suitable stretchers, splints, slings and emergency transport are available.
5. Where necessary, apply self-treatment immediately and as advised above. If response to self-treatment is not rapid,

always take professional advice from one of the recommended practitioners.

6. If in any doubt at all, never continue to play with an injury unless professional advice is available. Always take professional advice when making any decision as to whether or not to recommence playing after an injury.

If the above guidelines are followed, and the general and specific advice given in the preceding chapters of the book adhered to, then anybody should be able to enjoy their particular sport without any undue interference through lack of fitness, unnecessary injury or inefficient treatment of traumatic injuries sustained.

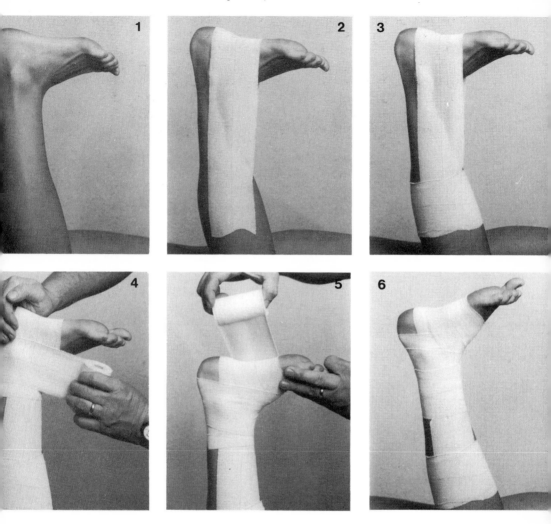

1. Ankle Strapping

Flex the foot with toes towards the leg as shown in picture 1. Next, place a stirrup of *Elastoplast* or similar bandage as shown in picture 2, with more tension on the side of the ankle which is most damaged. If the ankle is damaged on both sides, then the tension should be even. This stirrup is fixed to the leg with a circle of *Elastoplast*, as shown in picture 3, and then bound around the ankle with a figure-of-8 bandage, as shown in pictures 4 and 5, making sure that there are no wrinkles or creases in the tape as these can be uncomfortable. The strapping is then completed by running the *Elastoplast* a little way up the leg as shown in picture 6, and with this support the ankle is both comfortable and, in many cases, usable where it would be impossible without correct strapping.

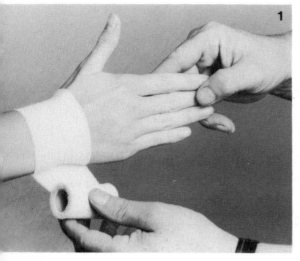
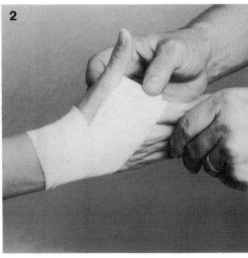
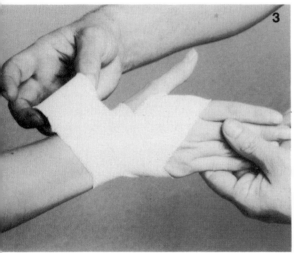
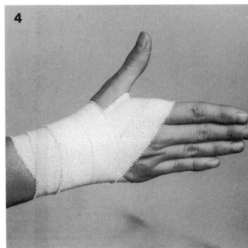

2. Wrist Strapping

Take the hand as shown in picture 1, with the thumb extended, and apply the first layer of tape around the damaged wrist in the direction illustrated. Take one layer of strapping between the thumb and forefinger and then back down the wrist as shown in pictures 2 and 3. The strapping is then completed as shown in picture 4. In case of serious wrist damage, added support can be gained by taking one or two more layers of strapping through the thumb while supporting the wrist.

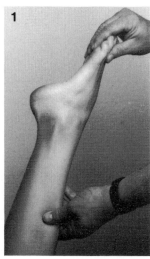
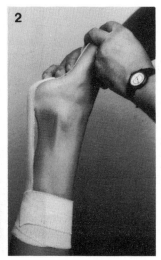
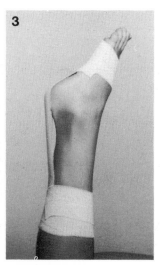

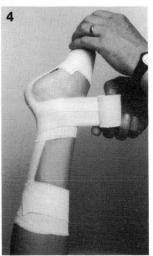
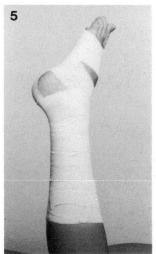

3. Achilles Strapping

Hold the leg with the foot pointed, as in picture 1, making sure that full stretch is achieved before applying the first strip of plaster as shown in picture 2. This should be attached to the top of the leg first, then stretched tightly down over the foot and fixed as in picture 3. The gap between the plaster and the ankle can clearly be seen: the plaster at this stage should be taut. The plaster is pulled tight to the back of the heel and the Achilles as in picture 4, then with one turn round the foot, the strapping is continued up to the supporting strap as shown in figure 5. This strapping is tremendously helpful where a strained or painful Achilles has been suffered and should be used if there is any tendency to pain around the Achilles when undergoing heavy physical exercise.

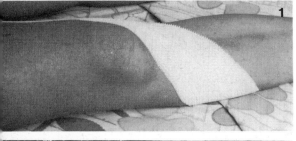

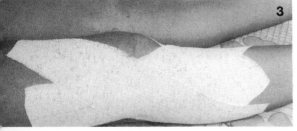

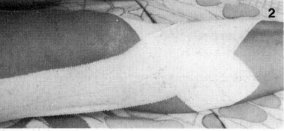

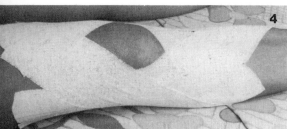

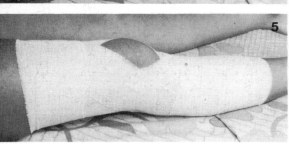

4. Knee Strapping

Knees are very vulnerable in many sports, and strain or damage is often suffered. With correct strapping, not only can discomfort be eased but, in many cases, sport can be undertaken quite safely without further damage occurring. Where persistent ligament problems have been suffered, strapping as illustrated permits participation without further risk of damage. Place the first strip of tape as shown in photograph 1, making sure that it is tight across the side of the knee. Place the second strip as in picture 2, again with good tension up the side of the knee. Another piece of tape is placed each side of the knee as in picture 3, and 4, once again making sure that it is tightly applied. The strips of tape are then firmly strapped top and bottom, as in picture 5. The resulting bandage (picture 6) not only supports the knee but allows free movement in the process. It is most important to make sure that the side strappings are kept tight throughout the operation.

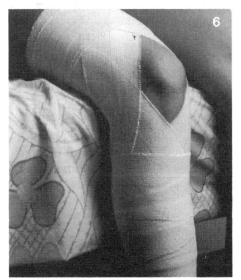

5. Thumb Strapping

The base thumb joint is particularly vulnerable to ligament damage in contact sports, and frequently needs strapping either as a short term measure whilst playing, or as a regular measure as a preventative to further damage. Once ligaments in the thumb have been put under severe stress, they can take a long time to repair, in which case the only way to ensure no further problems is correct support as illustrated. Take the hand as in picture 1, with the thumb extended, and take one turn of tape (of the size shown in picture 2) around the top of the thumb in the direction illustrated. This is then run across the gap between thumb and forefinger, as in picture 3, with a reasonable amount of tension placed upon it. The tape is taken under the wrist and back up towards the thumb as in picture 4, then pulled down into the base of the joint. Tighten the first strip of tape in the process, before turning round the thumb again as in picture 5. The tape is then taken round the wrist as in picture 6, back up between the thumb and forefinger as in picture 7, and taken lower down the thumb joint on the return strap as in picture 8. This ensures that the whole of the thumb is well supported, and the strapping is then run round the wrist as in picture 9 and back to the thumb as in pictures 10 and 11, to finish off with one last strap around the wrist as in picture 12. The finished strapping should offer complete support, as illustrated in pictures 13 and 14. If this strapping is used as support for playing, it restricts movement of the thumb to a range where no undue stress or strain is placed upon the major joint.

(Pictures continue overleaf.)

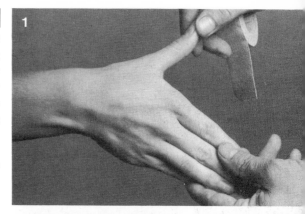

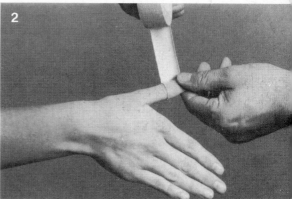

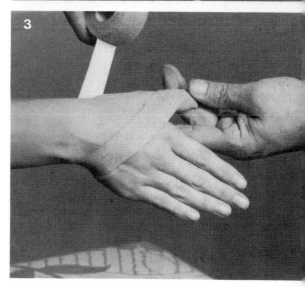

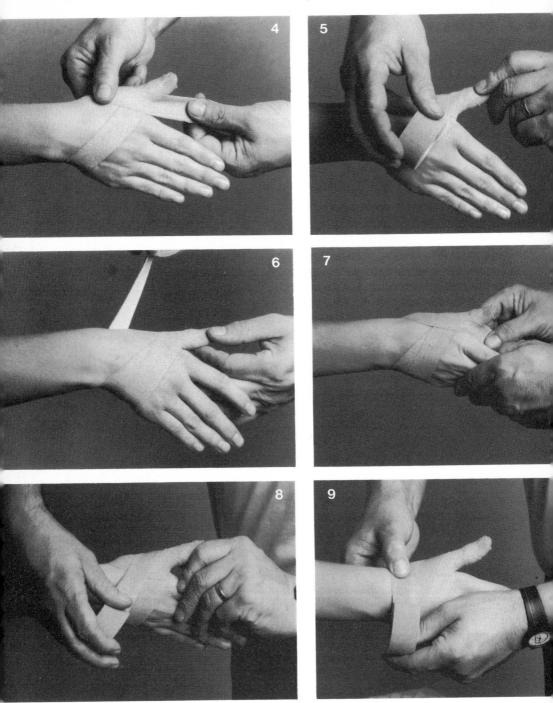

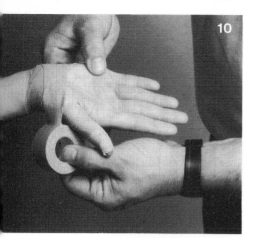

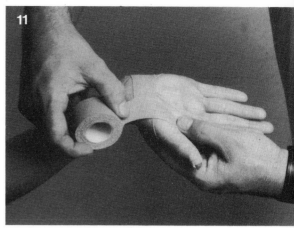

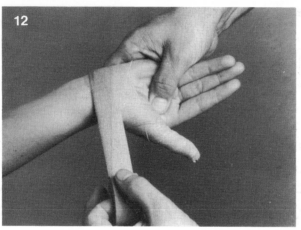

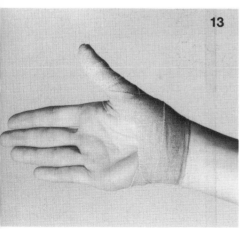

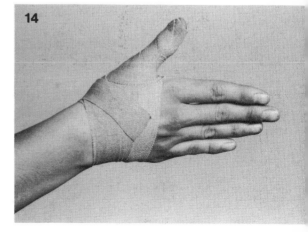

CONCLUSION

The pursuit of any form of sport is something which should be encouraged in everybody in the modern civilized world. Far too much time is spent in sedentary occupations and in stressful situations so that, unless some release is found and some means of stimulating body usage and breathing and circulation, then the general state of fitness of man as a whole will continue to decline.

By accepting the fact that health is a personal responsibility and by realizing that, in order to compete effectively and without danger in any sporting situation, a basic standard of health must be achieved, then not only will sport become a pleasure but the individual's quality of life will improve.

For sport to be the help it should be, everybody who undertakes it should look fitter, have less illness, and, above all, be a shining example in older age to all those who do not make the effort to involve themselves in a sporting situation. That in many cases people who have followed sport have serious illness problems and great difficulties in later life, underlines the need for the necessary self-discipline in the early stages. It is hoped that this book will give advice and encouragement to everybody who wants to lead a fuller and more satisfactory life.